Attachment-Informed Parent Coaching

Beth Troutman

Attachment-Informed Parent Coaching

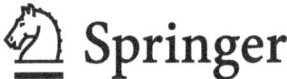 Springer

Beth Troutman
Department of Psychiatry
University of Iowa
Iowa City, IA, USA

ISBN 978-3-030-98569-1   ISBN 978-3-030-98570-7 (eBook)
https://doi.org/10.1007/978-3-030-98570-7

© The Editor(s) (if applicable) and The Author(s), under exclusive license to Springer Nature Switzerland AG 2022
This work is subject to copyright. All rights are solely and exclusively licensed by the Publisher, whether the whole or part of the material is concerned, specifically the rights of translation, reprinting, reuse of illustrations, recitation, broadcasting, reproduction on microfilms or in any other physical way, and transmission or information storage and retrieval, electronic adaptation, computer software, or by similar or dissimilar methodology now known or hereafter developed.
The use of general descriptive names, registered names, trademarks, service marks, etc. in this publication does not imply, even in the absence of a specific statement, that such names are exempt from the relevant protective laws and regulations and therefore free for general use.
The publisher, the authors and the editors are safe to assume that the advice and information in this book are believed to be true and accurate at the date of publication. Neither the publisher nor the authors or the editors give a warranty, expressed or implied, with respect to the material contained herein or for any errors or omissions that may have been made. The publisher remains neutral with regard to jurisdictional claims in published maps and institutional affiliations.

This Springer imprint is published by the registered company Springer Nature Switzerland AG
The registered company address is: Gewerbestrasse 11, 6330 Cham, Switzerland

In memory of my parents,
Betty McClure Troutman and Gary Troutman

Preface: Becoming an Attachment-Informed Parent Coach

Before diving into the details of how to coach parents from an attachment-informed perspective, I want to give you an idea of the *why*. Specifically, I want to give you an idea of my why—i.e., some of the experiences and relationships that shaped my development as an attachment-informed parent coach. How we are with the families we coach is as important as the specific techniques we use. How we are is informed by who we are and, like the families we serve, who we are is shaped by our relationships.

I decided to become a child psychologist at the beginning of the 1970s. My decision to become a clinical child psychologist who specialized in working with young children was influenced by my first job—babysitting two young girls in foster care when I was twelve years old. I loved that babysitting job. I especially loved playing with those two little girls. Of course, in hindsight, I wasn't much more than a child myself, but it didn't seem to me that I was at the time. I remember the two little girls inviting me into their play, imagining they were baby birds who were flying away from the nest. There was something especially poignant to me about these two young children pretending to be baby birds when I knew their own biological parents had failed to provide the support and nurturance they needed to confidently fly on their own.

At the same time I was forming relationships with these two young girls, I was forming a relationship with an author whose book would influence the path of my career, Richard D'Ambrosio, author of *No Language But a Cry* (1970). Although we think of relationships as being with the people we see in our lives on a regular basis, the powerful impact reading this book had on my career choice reminds me that not all formative relationships take place in person. Some of our formative relationships are with people we've never met—in my case, someone whom I knew only through his writing. It would be fifteen years before I would meet a child psychoanalyst in real life, but this book gave me the blueprint for the type of therapist I wanted to be when I grew up.

In *No Language But a Cry,* D'Ambrosio (1970) describes his psychoanalytic play therapy with a young girl—ironically, a twelve-year-old—who was mute following abuse and neglect by her parents. His description of how his therapeutic use of their relationship and of play allowed her to speak and to flourish had a profound impact on me when I was twelve. I decided then and there to become a clinical child psychologist and did not waver in my determination to pursue that path. I remember even not taking the career aptitude test offered at my high school because I was concerned the test results would not say child psychologist. If there is such a thing as imprinting in humans, I imprinted on D'Ambrosio after reading this book.

I recently reread *No Language But a Cry* (D'Ambrosio, 1970) for the first time in fifty years. I found it as touching as I did the first time I read it, and I realized that my twelve-year-old-self recognized in D'Ambrosio someone who saw the power of relationships—both in his own life and in what he brought to his work with children. Although my approach to working with young children has evolved since I read this book, I still recognize some of the core principles in the work I do today in D'Ambrosio's work.

In the 1970s and early 1980s, while working to complete my undergraduate and graduate degrees in psychology so I could pursue my dream of learning child psychoanalytic play therapy, I had additional experiences that ended up informing my approach to early-childhood intervention.

Sometimes our formative experiences are sought out—as in my decades-long quest to get trained in psychoanalytic play therapy—and at other times we get lucky. The formative experience I was lucky to have in graduate school at the University of Iowa in the 1980s was learning behavioral parent coaching from John Knutson. I learned to coach the parent of a highly disruptive three-year-old in strategies for managing her child's behavior. As I stood behind the one-way mirror coaching the parent through a bug in the ear, I remember thinking that this was not at all what I expected therapy to be like. It was certainly nothing like the psychoanalytic play therapy I'd read about when I decided to become a child psychologist. Instead of interacting with the child, I was coaching the parent while they interacted with the child. I also remember my nervousness about whether the technology would work, the excitement of seeing the child's behavior and relationship with his mother improve, and his mother's gratitude for help in addressing his behavior problems.

During graduate school, I also learned about Mary Ainsworth's research on attachment theory (Ainsworth, 1967, 1969; Ainsworth et al., 1978). After thousands of hours observing infants in their homes in Uganda and in Baltimore, Maryland, Mary Ainsworth developed the Strange Situation Procedure to demonstrate the balance between the attachment system and the exploratory system in babies (Ainsworth et al., 1978). The Strange Situation Procedure is a structured observation of parent-infant interactions involving brief separations and reunions between parent and baby. Conducting Strange Situation Procedures for my dissertation research hooked me on attachment theory and on the importance of observation in understanding parent-child relationships.

When observing mothers and babies together in the Strange Situation Procedure, I was struck by how these babies had learned strategies for being in relationships before they had language. In other words, in psychotherapy with my adult patients, I was talking about their relationships with others—i.e., their narrative memory. However, in the Strange Situation Procedure, I was seeing the power of procedural memory—what the baby had learned about how to function in relationships. Procedural memories are our "how to" memories—the automatic patterns of how to tie a shoe or how to ride a bike. Since patterns of attachment are developed before infants have language, they are also stored as "how to" memories—in this case how to be in relationship and how to communicate feelings to parents.

I learned psychoanalytic play therapy during my internship at the Yale Child Study Center from 1986 to 1987. There I saw how children's attachment experiences with their parents affected the children's interactions with me. In my consultations with the parents of children I was seeing in play therapy, I realized parents had their own set of "how to" memories that were developed before they could talk—experiences that affected their interactions with me and with their child.

I continued to study attachment theory as a faculty member at the University of Minnesota and the University of Iowa and to integrate concepts of attachment theory into my work with children and their parents (Caspers et al., 2005; Caspers et al., 2009; Caspers et al., 2007; Caspers et al., 2006; Troutman, 1992, 1998, 2002, 2003; Troutman et al., 1999, 2000, 2010; Troutman & Cardi, 1999; Troutman & Momany, 2012). As described in more detail in Chap. 2, after 20 years of studying attachment theory and psychoanalytic approaches, I returned to the behavioral parent coaching approach I had learned in graduate school.

When I began doing behavioral parent coaching again, I realized that my years of studying attachment theory had changed me. I had a new appreciation for the effectiveness of in vivo coaching with parents. Coaching a parent while they were playing with their child allowed me to observe the procedural memories guiding the parent-child interactions. I realized that I was in a unique position to help parents develop new strategies or "how to" memories as I supported them in responding in new ways to their child. Coaching parents to develop healthier, more effective strategies during their interactions with their child is the focus of this book. Those strategies are described in detail in the following chapters.

Iowa City, IA, USA   Beth Troutman

References

Ainsworth, M. (1967). *Infancy in Uganda*. Johns Hopkins Press.
Ainsworth, M. (1969). Object relations, dependency and attachment: A theoretical review of the infant-mother relationship. *Child Development, 40*, 969–1025.
Ainsworth, M., Blehar, M., Waters, E., & Wall, S. (1978). *Patterns of attachment: A psychological study of the Strange situation*. Erlbaum.
Caspers, K. M., Cadoret, R. J., Langbehn, D., Yucuis, R., & Troutman, B. (2005). Contributions of attachment style and perceived social support to lifetime use of illicit substances. *Addictive Behaviors, 30*(5), 1007–1011.

Caspers, K. M., Paradiso, S., Yucuis, R., Troutman, B., Arndt, S., & Philibert, R. (2009). Association between the serotonin transporter promoter polymorphism (5-HTTLPR) and adult unresolved attachment. *Development Psychology, 45*(1), 64–76.

Caspers, K. M., Yucuis, R., Troutman, B., Arndt, S., & Langbehn, D. (2007). A sibling adoption study of adult attachment: The influence of shared environment on attachment state of mind. *Attachment & Human Development, 9*(4), 375–391.

Caspers, K. M., Yucuis, R., Troutman, B., & Spinks, R. (2006). Attachment as an organizer of behavior: Implications for substance abuse problems and willingness to seek treatment. *Substance Abuse Treatment, Prevention, and Policy, 1*, 32.

D'Ambrosio, R. (1970). *No language but a cry*. Dell.

Troutman, B. (1992). Infant psychiatry. *Current Opinions in Psychiatry, 5*, 477–480.

Troutman, B. (1998). *Attachment in young foster children: Psychological and societal considerations*. Paper presented at the Department of Psychiatry Grand Rounds, University of Iowa College of Medicine.

Troutman, B. (2002). *Early childhood mental health: Models of prevention and early intervention*. Paper presented at the The Iowa Federation of the Council for Exceptional Children Spring conference, Ames, IA.

Troutman, B. (2003). *Meeting the needs of young children in foster care: Evidence-based models of assessment and intervention*. Paper presented at the The Fourth Annual Ohio Association for Infant Mental Health (OAIMH) Conference. Back from the Edge: Relationship-based interventions, Columbus, OH.

Troutman, B., Arndt, S., Caspers, K. M., & Yucuis, R. (2010). *Infant negative emotionality moderates the association between quantity of nonfamilial day care and infant-mother attachment*. Paper presented at the 57th Annual Meeting of the American Academy of Child & Adolescent Psychiatry, New York, NY.

Troutman, B., & Cardi, M. (1999). Barriers to the development of healthy attachments among young foster children. *Zero to Three, 19*(2), 33–34.

Troutman, B., Cardi, M., & Ryan, S. (1999). Infants placed in out-of-home care: Implications for attachment. *The Source, 9*(3), 12–15.

Troutman, B., & Momany, A. (2012). Use of selective serotonin reuptake inhibitors during pregnancy and disorganised infant-mother attachment. *Journal of Reproductive and Infant Psychology, 30*(3), 261–277.

Troutman, B., Ryan, S., & Cardi, M. (2000). The effects of foster care placement on young children's mental health. *Protecting Children, 16*(1), 30–34.

Acknowledgments

When my book *Integrating Behaviorism and Attachment Theory* was published in 2015, it felt like the end of a journey. I didn't realize that it was the end of one journey and the beginning of another. Thanks to Garth Heller from Springer for launching this new journey by suggesting I write a second book; discussing book ideas over lunch in New York made me feel like a writer. Thank you to Judy Jones and Olivia Ramya Chitranjan from Springer for accompanying me on this new journey. I appreciate your interest, encouragement, and patience as completing *Attachment-Informed Parent Coaching* became my pandemic project.

Many of the people who accompanied me on my previous journey also accompanied me on the journey to writing *Attachment-Informed Parent Coaching*. Thank you for being my friends and allies in improving services for families. You continue to inspire and challenge me.

Thank you to my friend, Betsy Momany, for your friendship and support since graduate school and your work to improve healthcare services for children and their families. Thanks to the fabulous group of friends who currently provide training in IoWA-PCIT: Samantha Byrns, Stacie Daily, Kami Guzman-Milligan, Joanna Halbur, Julie Mertz, Allison Momany, Katie Obert, Bre-Ann Slay, Nikki Van Ginkel, and Tracy Vozar. Thank you for making IoWA-PCIT your own, your passion for improving the lives of children, and for continuing to move forward in applying attachment theory to work with children and families.

Thank you to my friend and former student, Lea Boldt, for doing brilliant research on attachment, asking challenging questions, and helping me build a snowman. Thank you to my friend and former student, Burgundy Johnson, for reminding me how much fun it is to do parent coaching and for your compassionate work with families. Thank you to my friend and former student, Allison Momany, for your long-term support and enthusiasm for IoWA-PCIT, your help with research, and for describing IoWA-PCIT as being like a hot fudge sundae.

Thank you to my friend and writing coach, Mary Allen. I feel like I first met you in the Coralville library when I began reading your book, *Rooms of Heaven*. Your beautiful, vivid prose continues to be a model for the writer I want to be when I grow up. Thank you for helping me become a better writer and for believing in this book.

Thank you to my friends, Marta Shinn and Arlene Turner, for inspiring me to incorporate more active play into my life; your joy in movement started a journey that influenced the final chapter of this book. Thank you to my friend and somatic movement therapist, Meg Eginton, for teaching me about the role of movement in healing, providing a place to dance, and discussing object relations theories with me. Thank you for asking me how children in different attachment relationships dance, a question I tried to answer in the final chapter.

Thank you to my friend, colleague, former student, and former boss, Tracy Vozar, for your decades-long support. Special thanks for being my writing partner and co-teaching with me at the University of Denver. The opportunity to see IoWA-PCIT through your eyes and the eyes of your students kept me motivated while working on this book. I hope your students enjoy reading this book as much as you think they will.

Thank you to my friend, Tania Cargo, for our numerous and wide-ranging discussions. I continue to learn from you. Thank you for your interest and support in integrating attachment principles into PCIT and your drive to improve interventions for families. The opportunity to spend time with you, your trainees, and your family in New Zealand in February, 2020, was a source of inspiration as I worked on this book. Also, the opportunity to spend an evening with you and Denise Guy discussing attachment helped me think through the core components of attachment-informed work with families.

Thank you to my friend, Kelly Pelzel, for always being available to answer questions or bounce ideas off. I'm amazed at what we can resolve in a coffee break. Being able to talk with you about different models of parent coaching, attachment, movement, and object relations helped me clarify what I wanted to communicate in this book. Thank you for finding the perfect epigraph for the last chapter and for being an early, enthusiastic reader.

Thank you to John Knutson for teaching me behavioral parent coaching. Thank you to Cheryl McNeil for teaching me how to disseminate PCIT and how to savor the joy of parent coaching. Thank you to Dymphna van den Boom for teaching me attachment coaching for irritable infants. Thank you to Kent Hoffman, Bert Powell, and Glen Cooper for teaching me Circle of Security.

Thank you to Alan and June Sroufe for coding Infant Strange Situation Procedures for my research on irritable infants. Thank you to Alan Sroufe and Betty Carlson for teaching me about infant attachment. Thank you to June Sroufe for teaching me about the Adult Attachment Interview (AAI). Thank you to Remi Cadoret and Kristen Caspers for the opportunity to learn to code the AAI and be involved in research on adult attachment.

Thank you to Ellen Moss and Vanessa Lecompte for coding Preschool Strange Situation Procedures for my research on IoWA-PCIT. Thank you to Ellen Moss, Jean-Francois Bureau, and Audrey-Ann Deneault for teaching me about preschool attachment.

Acknowledgments

Thank you to Tanager Place for funding research on IoWA-PCIT. Your commitment to funding local initiatives and your support of IoWA-PCIT research and training is a model for bridging the science to service gap. Thank you to the University of Iowa Department of Psychiatry for pilot funding to improve my expertise in coding preschool attachment. Thank you to the University of Denver for the opportunity to do a visiting professorship in 2021. Learning from the faculty and students in the Graduate School of Professional Psychology while working on this book provided intellectual stimulation and moral support when I most needed it. A special thank you to the staff and students at the Caring for You & Baby (CUB) clinic. You were in my mind often when writing this book. Thank you to the staff at the Nebraska Resource Project for Vulnerable Young Children at the University of Nebraska Lincoln for your support of IoWA-PCIT training and your advocacy for young children.

Thanks to the families who have participated in my research on IoWA-PCIT and let me coach them in new ways to interact. Each one of you has taught me about attachment, parent coaching, and myself. You are the reason I do this work.

Thank you to my husband, Ralph Johnson, for being my secure base and safe haven. I can't think of anyone I would rather weather a pandemic with.

Contents

1	**Born for Relationships**	1
	Introduction	1
	Born to Connect	2
	Born to Help	4
	Attachment Priming in Children	5
	Patterns of Attachment	6
	The Bottom Line	7
	References	8
2	**The IoWA-PCIT Parent Coaching Model**	9
	Behavioral Parent Coaching	9
	Development of the IoWA-PCIT Parent Coaching Model	10
	The IoWA-PCIT Model	12
	Research on IoWA-PCIT	14
	Parenting Factors Associated with Disruptive Behavior	14
	Outcome Studies	15
	Clinical Experience	15
	Training in IoWA-PCIT	16
	The Bottom Line	16
	References	16
3	**How to Complete an Attachment-Informed Early-Childhood Mental Health Assessment**	19
	Understanding Problems in a Relationship Context	19
	Goals of Attachment-Informed Assessment	20
	What Parents of Infants and Young Children Need from Therapists	20
	Parent's Working Models of Attachment	21
	Initial Intake	23
	Pretreatment Assessment for IoWA-PCIT	24
	Attachment Assessment (Preschool Strange Situation Procedure)	25
	Behavioral Assessment (Dyadic Parent–Child Interaction Coding System)	25

	Clues to Parent's Working Model of Attachment	26
	The Bottom Line	29
	References	29
4	**How to Coach Parents to Follow Their Child's Lead in Play**	**31**
	Born to Play	31
	Benefits of Child-Led Play with a Parent	32
	Child-Directed Interaction (CDI)	32
	CDI Engage and Teach Session	33
	What Parents Need from Therapists During the CDI Engage and Teach Session	34
	Parent Verbalizations Used During CDI	34
	Behavior Description	35
	Reflection	35
	Labeled Praise	35
	Concerns About Praise	36
	Parent Nonverbal Behaviors Used During CDI	37
	Imitation	37
	Enjoy	37
	Parent Verbalizations Avoided During CDI	38
	Criticism	38
	Commands	38
	Questions	39
	Managing Behavior Problems During CDI	39
	Differential Attention	40
	Stopping CDI	40
	CDI Homework	40
	Managing Child's Behavior Outside of CDI	41
	CDI Coaching	42
	What Parents Need from Therapists During CDI Coaching	42
	Tracking Progress in CDI	42
	Parent Ratings of Disruptive Behavior	43
	Observations of Parent–Child Interactions	43
	Coaching CDI in the Family's Home	44
	Determining How Long to Continue the CDI Phase	45
	The Bottom Line	45
	References	46
5	**How to Coach Parents to Set Limits and Improve Child Compliance**	**47**
	Parent-Directed Interaction (PDI)	47
	Importance of Limit-Setting in Healthy Attachment	48
	Research on Limit-Setting and Secure Attachment	49
	Eight Rules of Effective Commands in PDI	50
	Positively State the Command	50
	Reason Before Command and/or After Compliance	51

	Age-Appropriate Command	51
	Calm and Courteous Command	52
	Tell, Don't Ask	52
	Individual Command	53
	Clear Command	53
	Enough Commands	53
	Response to Compliance	54
	Response to Noncompliance	54
	Response to Getting Off Time-Out Chair and Unsafe Behavior on Time-Out Chair	56
	Explaining PDI to the Child: Coaching Parent Through Explanation	57
	Explaining PDI to the Child: Therapist Explanation	59
	Initial In-Session PDI Commands	59
	Play Commands	59
	Real Commands	60
	In-Session Balance Between PDI and CDI	60
	Tracking Progress in PDI	61
	PDI Rollout	61
	The Bottom Line	61
	References	62
6	**How to Tailor Parent Coaching: Four Examples**	63
	Tailoring and Adaptations of Traditional PCIT	63
	Why to Tailor IoWA-PCIT to Working Models of Attachment	64
	Example # 1: Isabella	65
	Example #2: John	66
	Example #3: Rhonda	68
	Example #4: Hank	70
	The Bottom Line	71
	References	72
7	**Ordinary Magic: How to Tailor Coaching for Dyads with Secure Attachment**	73
	How to Recognize Secure Child–Parent Attachment	73
	How to Recognize Secure Attachment in Infant Strange Situation Procedure	74
	Comparison of Strange Situation Procedure in Infants and Preschool-Aged Children	75
	How to Recognize Secure Attachment in Preschool Strange Situation Procedure	76
	Development of Secure Child–Parent Attachment	76
	Attachment Signals	76
	Sensitive Responsiveness to Attachment Signals	77
	How Secure Attachment May Be Adaptive for the Child	78
	Prevalence of Secure Attachment Pattern	78

How to Promote Secure Attachment: Coaching Parents
To Be More Sensitively Responsive to Attachment Signals.......... 79
How to Promote Secure Attachment in Infants................... 80
How to Promote Secure Attachment in Toddlers
and Preschool-Aged Children................................ 81
Course of IoWA-PCIT with Secure Dyads....................... 81
The Bottom Line.. 82
References... 82

8 Open to Change: How to Tailor Coaching for Parents with Secure/Autonomous Attachment......................... 85
How to Recognize Parents' Secure/Autonomous
Working Model of Attachment................................ 85
How to Recognize Earned Secure Working Model of Attachment..... 86
How Secure/Autonomous Attachment May Be Adaptive............ 86
Prevalence of Secure/Autonomous Attachment 88
Course of IoWA-PCIT with Secure/Autonomous Parents 88
Course of IoWA-PCIT with Earned Secure Parents 88
The Bottom Line.. 89
References... 90

9 Can't Live with You, Can't Live Without You: How to Tailor Coaching for Dyads with Ambivalent/Resistant Attachment 91
How to Recognize Ambivalent/Resistant Pattern of Attachment 91
Development of Ambivalent/Resistant Attachment Pattern 92
How Ambivalent/Resistant Attachment
May Be Adaptive for the Child................................ 94
Prevalence of Ambivalent/Resistant Attachment Pattern 94
How to Promote Secure Attachment in Ambivalent/Resistant Dyads .. 94
Course of IoWA-PCIT with Ambivalent/Resistant Dyads 96
Countertransference/Common Pitfalls 97
The Bottom Line.. 97
References... 97

10 Mired in Relationships: How to Tailor Coaching for Parents with Preoccupied Attachment 99
How to Recognize Preoccupied Working Model
of Attachment in Parents..................................... 99
How Preoccupied Working Model May Be Adaptive 100
Prevalence of Preoccupied Attachment 100
Course of IoWA-PCIT with Preoccupied Parents 100
Countertransference/Common Pitfalls........................... 103
Preoccupied Parent in a Secure Relationship with Their Child 107
Preoccupied Parent in an Avoidant Relationship with Their Child 107
The Bottom Line.. 107
References 108

Contents

**11 Going It Alone: How to Tailor Coaching for Dyads
with Avoidant Attachment** 109
How to Recognize Avoidant Pattern of Attachment 109
Prevalence of Avoidant Attachment 110
Development of Avoidant Attachment 110
How Avoidant Attachment May Be Adaptive for the Child 111
How to Promote Secure Attachment in Avoidant Dyads 111
Course of IoWA-PCIT with Avoidant Dyads 112
The Bottom Line 113
References 113

**12 What Does Not Kill Me Makes Me Stronger:
How to Tailor Coaching for Parents with Dismissing Attachment** ... 115
How to Recognize Dismissing Attachment 115
How Dismissing Attachment May Be Adaptive 116
Prevalence of Dismissing Attachment 117
Course of IoWA-PCIT with Dismissing Parents 117
Dismissing Parent in a Secure Relationship with Their Child 120
Dismissing Parent in an Ambivalent/Resistant Relationship
with Their Child 120
The Bottom Line 121
References 121

**13 Attachment Anxiety: How to Tailor Coaching
for Dyads with Disorganized and Controlling Attachment** 123
Role of Loss in Disorganized Attachment 124
Role of Parents' Frightening Behavior
in Disorganized/Disoriented Attachment 125
Role of Parents' Frightened Behavior
in Disorganized/Disoriented Attachment 125
How to Recognize Disorganized/Disoriented Attachment 126
How to Recognize Disorganized/Controlling Attachment 126
Development of Controlling Attachment 127
How Disorganized/Disoriented Attachment
May Be Adaptive for the Child 128
How Controlling Attachment May Be Adaptive for the Child 129
Prevalence of Disorganized/Disoriented Attachment 129
Prevalence of Controlling Attachment 129
Course of IoWA-PCIT with Disorganized/Disoriented
and Controlling Attachment Relationships 130
The Bottom Line 132
References 133

**14 Ghosts in the Playroom: How to Tailor Coaching
for Parents with Unresolved Attachment Loss or Trauma** 135
How to Recognize Unresolved Attachment Loss or Trauma 135
Development of Unresolved Attachment 136

	How Unresolved Attachment May Be Adaptive.	136
	Interventions Associated with Resolution of Unresolved Attachment	136
	Prevalence of Unresolved Attachment	138
	Course of Treatment with Parents with Unresolved Attachment	138
	The Bottom Line.	140
	References	141
15	**Attachment Trauma: How to Tailor Coaching for Parents of Children in Foster Care**	**143**
	Challenges Faced by Young Children in Foster Care	143
	Attachment Myth That Damages Young Children in Foster Care	144
	How Early Attachment Trauma Impacts Attachment Relationships	145
	Helping Young Children Heal from Attachment Trauma	146
	Challenges Faced by Foster Parents	146
	Child-Directed Interaction (CDI) with Foster Parents	148
	Parent-Directed Interaction (PDI) with Foster Parents.	149
	Working with Biological Parents of Young Children in Foster Care	151
	When Attachment-Informed Parent Coaching with Biological Parents of Children in Foster Care Is Not Appropriate	151
	Working with Older Children and Adolescents in Foster Care	152
	The Bottom Line.	153
	References	153
16	**Adoption and Attachment: How to Tailor Coaching for Parents of Adopted Children**	**155**
	Attachment and Adoption.	156
	Working with Adopted Children and Their Parents	156
	The Bottom Line.	158
	References	159
17	**Behind the Mirror: Learning and Growing as an Attachment-Informed Therapist**	**161**
	Growing as an Attachment-Informed Therapist	161
	How Therapists' Working Models of Attachment Impact Their Communication with Patients.	162
	What Secure Therapists Sound Like When Communicating with Their Patients	163
	What Dismissing Therapists Sound Like When Communicating with Their Patients	164
	What Preoccupied Therapists Sound Like When Communicating with Their Patients	165
	Disorganizing Moments in Parent Coaching	166
	What I've Learned from Coaching Parents with Different Working Models of Attachment	166
	What I've Learned from Working with Secure Dyads	167

	What I've Learned from Working with Avoidant Dyads	167
	What I've Learned from Working with Ambivalent/Resistant Dyads	167
	What I've Learned from Working with Disorganized and Controlling Dyads	168
	The Bottom Line	168
	References	168
18	**Dancing Toward Security: Adding New Steps to Your Attachment Dance**	**171**
	The Power of Dance	171
	Dance as a Coping Strategy During the COVID-19 Pandemic	172
	Virtual Dance Parties	172
	Sing.Play.Love.® Parties	173
	BeMoved® Dance Classes	173
	Born to Dance	174
	Movement and Attachment	174
	Movement in Secure Dyads	175
	Movement in Ambivalent/Resistant Dyads	175
	Movement in Avoidant Dyads	176
	Movement in Disorganized Dyads	176
	Movement in Controlling Dyads	176
	Providing Opportunities to Dance	177
	Dance Music	177
	Songs for Secure Pattern of Attachment and Secure/Autonomous State of Mind	178
	Songs for Avoidant Pattern of Attachment and Dismissing State of Mind	179
	Songs for Ambivalent/Resistant Pattern of Attachment and Preoccupied State of Mind	180
	Songs for Disorganized Pattern of Attachment and Unresolved State of Mind	181
	Song for Controlling–Punitive Attachment	182
	Song for Controlling–Caregiving Attachment	182
	The Bottom Line	183
	References	183
Index		**185**

Chapter 1
Born for Relationships

This chapter describes the theoretical foundation for using a relationship-based parent coaching approach to address emotional and behavioral difficulties in young children. I discuss humans' biological predisposition for relationships and review seminal research on attachment theory and altruism.

Introduction

This book is for early-childhood interventionists who work with parents to address children's emotional and behavioral difficulties. At its core, this book is about the healing power of relationships. It is about the special relationship parents have with their children—as well as the incumbent stress and anxiety that comes with that relationship. It is also about the special relationship that early-childhood interventionists have with parents and children. This book reflects the history of my relationships—the imprint left by the relationships that guide my work with families. Although the principles of attachment theory can be applied across the life span, this book is geared toward therapists who are interested in using an attachment-informed parent coaching approach to address problems of infants, toddlers, and preschool-aged children.

Language is a necessary but imprecise tool for communicating about relationships. A brief note about the language I use to describe the caregivers who help young children develop and thrive follows. Throughout this book, I have chosen to use the term parent to describe the various members of a child's social network who provide physical and emotional caretaking for a child. Parents might include biological parents, foster parents, stepparents, grandparents, great-grandparents, aunts, uncles, older siblings, and/or childcare providers. The term "psychological parent" (Goldstein, Solnit, Goldstein, & Freud, 1996; Robertson & Robertson, 1989) or "alloparent" (Hrdy, 1999) has sometimes been used in the literature to distinguish between biological parents and other important attachment figures. I have chosen to keep the focus on defining a parent from the perspective of the child—the person who the child depends on for care.

Therapist is the term I have chosen to describe the individuals this book is targeted to—that is, early-childhood interventionists who want to incorporate attachment-informed parent coaching into their work with young children and their parents. While attachment-informed parent coaching is a specific approach to addressing problems in young children, we are therapists first and foremost. We bring our therapeutic skills in building relationships with distressed individuals to the very important work of building relationships with a distressed child and the child's distressed parents. My favorite title was given to me by a young play therapy patient who referred to me as her "feelings Doctor." But, in fact, I am an "attachment Doctor." My hope is this book will help you on your path to becoming the type of therapist you want to be as you learn about how to incorporate attachment-informed parent coaching into your work.

The young children who are referred for early-childhood intervention present with a variety of concerns related to the myriad of tasks involved in growing into a fully functioning human. Parents often describe problems that significantly strain the parent–child relationship—for example, aggression toward the parent, failure to follow directions, and separation anxiety. The parents who seek our help because of vexing early-childhood issues bring their own set of beliefs and challenges based on their early experiences.

When therapists are faced with the challenging behaviors and problematic interactions that bring parents to seek help, there can be a tendency to forget that we are born to be in relationships. Perhaps, this is why I find attachment theory so compelling: it reminds me that we are born to connect. In addition, understanding the development of healthy child–parent attachment gives me a road map for helping parents and children find their way to more positive interactions.

Early in my career, an observant student commented that I looked forward to new issues of *Child Development* the way she looked forward to new issues of *Vogue*. This is an apt description of my excitement about developmental research. While parenting and therapy fads have come and gone over the course of my career, the research on attachment theory has steadily grown. In this chapter, I share what I consider some of the timeless lessons of research on attachment theory.

Born to Connect

Attachment theory grew out of an attempt to explain what it is that makes us uniquely human. John Bowlby, a child psychiatrist who is considered the father of attachment theory, sought to understand how a child's experiences with his or her parents influenced the child's development (Bowlby, 1958, 1959, 1960, 1969, 1973, 1980). He was especially interested in understanding the biological basis of the profound influence of early experiences with parents on social-emotional development. His work was strongly influenced by ethologists who studied innate aspects of caregiving in animals (i.e., instinct).

Bowlby's colleague, Mary Ainsworth, is considered the mother of attachment theory (Ainsworth, 1967; Ainsworth, Blehar, Waters, & Wall, 1978). Mary Ainsworth was a psychologist who conducted empirical studies based on Bowlby's theories. The data from these studies provided support and, in some cases, modifications to the theory. Thus, from its initial conception, attachment theory was a data-led theory.

As described by Bowlby and Ainsworth, attachment theory explains the unique sociability of humans and the need for infants and young children to interact with and receive attention from their primary caregivers. Ainsworth noted that both social learning theory and psychoanalytic theory had a "cupboard love" view of the interactions between young children and their parents (Ainsworth, 1969). That is, those theories concluded that infants and young children became attached to their parents because of the material comforts provided by the parents—for example, food.

In the language of behaviorism, food was considered a primary reinforcer, while attention and comfort were not. The classic studies by American psychologist Harry Harlow indicated this idea was erroneous (Harlow, 1958; Suomi, van der Horst, & van der Veer, 2008). In one of Harlow's early studies, he gave young chimpanzees two "substitute mothers" (Harlow, 1958). One of these substitute mothers was made of wire and had a bottle through which the baby chimp could get nourishment. The other substitute mother was made out of cloth but offered no nourishment, at least not nourishment of the food variety. Harlow's (1958) study showed that baby chimps went to the cloth mother instead of the wire mother, seeking comfort over food, especially during times of stress—just as Bowlby had predicted. The videos of these early Harlow experiments are profoundly disturbing for precisely the reason they demonstrated—they highlight the need for comfort from a parent. The "wire mother" is a term that resonates with people who had their physical needs but not their emotional needs met by their parents.

Two other individuals whose work was essential to the development of attachment theory were James and Joyce Robertson (Robertson & Robertson, 1989). The Robertsons were trained as psychoanalytic social workers and were colleagues of both John Bowlby and Anna Freud. One of James Robertson's most important contributions to attachment theory was delineating the stages young children go through when separated from their parents without adequate support from an alternative, responsive caregiver. The stages documented by James Robertson of young children separated from their parents were protest, despair, and detachment (Robertson, 1953). In the protest phase, young children cried and reached for their parents, protesting the separation. In the despair phase, young children seemed to give up, turning away from interactions with others when separated from their parents. In the detachment phase, young children no longer seemed interested in interacting with their parents when reunited with their parents.

Humans are uniquely social and especially dependent on relationships. Compared to other mammals, baby humans are unusually inept at birth. They are unable to walk, unable to defend themselves, and unable to forage for their food. One of

Bowlby's early observations about the unique strengths and vulnerabilities of young children is that they seek a person rather than a place when they are distressed. That propensity has led to the success of the human species. But it also places us in a position of being uniquely vulnerable to the primary caregivers we rely on to take care of us.

Since attachment relationships are so critical to survival, it makes sense to place them at the center of our efforts to address early-childhood mental health problems. It reminds us that even in profoundly disturbed parent–child relationships, there is a need to be in relationship. This need can be the source of psychopathology, but it can be the source of healing as well. Because of the inborn instinct for attachment, we are working with the evolutionary heritage of humans when we approach problems from the perspective of attachment theory. We are born to be in relationships with others. By helping remove barriers to healthy attachment relationships, we can address difficulties and improve both the parent's and child's functioning.

The first step in harnessing the innate desire for relationships in our therapeutic work with children and their families is to recognize it. Just knowing that evolution has made us biologically prepared for attachment relationships has impacted my approach to working with children and parents. It gave me hope to know I was working with our innate characteristics. It helped me begin to recognize that the need for attachment was still there even when those needs were not being met. Keeping in mind the innate human desire for relationships also helps us understand the factors that promote feelings of attachment. This is a strength-based approach that builds on children's and parents' positive intentions to be in relationship—even when they engage in maladaptive ways to maintain these relationships. Factors that promote positive attachment feelings and behaviors can be effective even in the face of previous negative attachment experiences.

Born to Help

Parents want their children to engage in prosocial behaviors—for example, sharing and being helpful. Research by Warneken and Tomasello (2006) opened my eyes to the extent to which young children are hardwired to be helpful. Like attachment, altruism turns out to be part of our evolutionary heritage.

When you think about what it takes to be altruistic, it involves both cognitive and moral development. You have to first perceive the other person's need and then take action to meet that need. This is best illustrated by my favorite example from Warneken and Tomasello's (2006) study of altruism. One of the videos accompanying the article shows a petite 18-month-old girl standing shyly next to her mother as a tall adult male enters the room. She watches intently from her mother's side as the male struggles to put away a stack of magazines in a cabinet with closed doors. After watching his struggle, with no apparent cue from her mother, she toddles over to the cabinet, opens the doors for him, and looks up at him. The entire sequence of events takes about 30 seconds. But it communicates a great deal about the capacity for altruism already present at 18 months of age. In a series of contrived situations like this, Warneken and Tomasello (2006) demonstrated repeatedly the tendency of young humans to spontaneously and voluntarily help an unrelated adult who was struggling with a task. The vast majority of the young children in this study (more than 90%) helped in at least one of the situations where someone needed assistance. The chimpanzees also displayed altruism in similar situations but at a lower rate than human infants.

Attachment Priming in Children

Attachment theory suggests that the inborn need to be in relationship and care for others can be activated or deactivated depending on cues from the environment. One of the reasons there is such a variety of ways to be in relationship is we are an adaptable species—a species that can survive in harsh environments where it pays to compete for limited resources and a species that can survive in environments where there are benefits to cooperation.

The activation of the attachment system by using specific cues is called attachment security priming. In a simple but brilliant example of priming, 18-month-olds were shown pictures of two dolls facing each other (the attachment prime), two dolls facing away from each other, or stacks of blocks (Over & Carpenter, 2009). The young children who were shown the two dolls facing each other were twice as likely to be altruistic in helping a stranger with a task following the attachment prime. Just the sight of two dolls facing each other gave the young toddlers enough of an attachment prime to lead to more altruism. It is as though this brief reminder of the importance of connection activated the part of our inheritance that reminded them of a world where there are benefits to cooperation.

Another example of the power of attachment priming is research by Brandi Stupica and her colleagues of 6-year-olds (Stupica, Brett, Woodhouse, & Cassidy, 2019). In this study, the attachment prime was pictures of mothers and children engaged in positive interactions. Following the prime, the children were shown stressful pictures of animal attacks, designed to evoke physiological responses—the fight or flight response characterized at the physiological level by shallow breathing, clammy palms, and a racing heart. Stupica et al. (2019) found that the simple attachment prime of showing children pictures of mothers and children engaged in positive interactions, before showing them the stressful pictures, led the children to be less physiologically reactive to the stressful pictures. This study demonstrates that seeing positive images of attachment reduces the response to stress—not just at a psychological level but at a physiological level.

One of the important lessons of attachment priming is that tapping into our inborn need for connection is an important source of healing, regardless of our previous experience with relationships. One of the aspects of the Stupica et al. (2019) study I found somewhat surprising was that the attachment priming reduced the physiological response to stress even for the children whose expectations regarding attachment relationships were more negative than positive. Prior to reading this study, I had wondered about the wisdom of displaying pictures of parents and children enjoying each other's company in clinics where the focus is improving parent–child interactions. These results suggest that not only is it not upsetting for troubled dyads to see models of parent–child interactions that are different from what they're experiencing, it is soothing and potentially helpful to them. Perhaps seeing the capacity for positive relationships helps them recognize that capacity in themselves.

Attachment theory gives us a way of conceptualizing what is important in parent–child relationships. To put it one way, it helps us focus on the signal instead of the noise in our work with families. It's easy for therapists to get hung up on what I call the noise—details such as whether parents use time-outs or co-sleep with their children. Attachment theory helps us focus on the signal—the quality of the relationship between the parents and the child. There are so many different ideas about what is important in parenting, as indicated by the large number of books on the market about how to parent. Yet, attachment theory has learned that what is important to being a good parent is consistent across cultures. And this can be studied and taught.

Patterns of Attachment

Because of the powerful need to be in relationship with their parents, infants learn early on how to get their attachment needs met given the limitations of their environment and their parents. These strategies are called patterns of attachment (Ainsworth et al., 1978). The majority of child–parent relationships fall into what is referred to as the secure pattern of attachment. Secure relationships have been described as "ordinary magic" (Masten, 2001) because they are so common we take them for granted, but they have a special place in protecting children from the inevitable challenges and stresses associated with growing up.

A securely attached child strikes a balance between relying on others and relying on themselves. Insecure attachment, the type of attachment that is a risk factor for a variety of emotional and behavioral problems, involves a lack of balance. That is, in an insecure attachment relationship the child's anxiety about getting their attachment needs met is reflected by putting too much emphasis on either exploration or relationships.

Too much emphasis on achievement and exploration is a type of insecure attachment referred to as avoidant attachment. Young children with an avoidant attachment to their parents often seem extremely competent. In fact, early researchers questioned the characterization of avoidant attachment as a risk factor due to these infants' apparent ability to easily handle separations from their parent and their focus on mastering the environment. Infants in an avoidant attachment relationship appear unfazed by their parent's return after a brief separation from them. Instead, when the parent comes back, the child turns to a toy and continues to play,

Table 1.1 Characteristics of avoidant, secure, and ambivalent/resistant attachment

Insecure avoidant	Secure	Insecure ambivalent/resistant
Focus on independence	Balance between attachment and exploration	Focus on relationship
Minimization of distress	Openly expresses distress	Heightening of distress

seemingly more focused on mastering the environment than on their relationship with their parent.

Too much emphasis on the relationship with the parent is a type of insecure attachment referred to as ambivalent/resistant attachment. At times it has also been referred to as anxious attachment. Infants in ambivalent/resistant attachment relationships are so focused on their parent that they are unable to explore the environment. They are extremely distressed when separated from their parent yet fail to be soothed by the presence of their parent. The characteristics of secure, avoidant, and ambivalent/resistant patterns of attachment are summarized in Table 1.1.

Mary Ainsworth's student, Mary Main, identified another type of insecure attachment that she called disorganized/disoriented attachment (Main & Solomon, 1990). In this type of attachment relationship, the parent is both the source of comfort and the source of anxiety, placing the child between a rock and a hard place. In disorganized/disoriented attachment, there is a momentary breakdown in the attachment strategy. The infant may show misdirected movements—for example, moving toward the mother at reunion only to abruptly change direction and move away. Or the infant may briefly appear disoriented—for example, freezing in place briefly with a dazed expression.

Later chapters provide more details on how to recognize secure, avoidant, ambivalent/resistant, and disorganized attachment. These "how to" chapters also provide information on how to help parents develop more balanced, secure relationships with their children while enhancing their child's social-emotional development.

The Bottom Line

Research on our biological predisposition for attachment tells us that we are working with rather than against the tide when we work to improve parent–child relationships. Or, as Selma Fraiberg said, working to improve parent–child interactions is "a little bit like having God on your side" (Osofsky, 1988). The fact that part of being uniquely human is being born for relationships means that young children and their parents are highly motivated to improve the quality of their relationships. And, when the relationship improves, there is a cascading effect that leads to improvement in other areas as well. It means that focusing our efforts on the quality of the relationship will benefit numerous aspects of child and parent functioning.

References

Ainsworth, M. (1967). *Infancy in Uganda*. Johns Hopkins Press.
Ainsworth, M. (1969). Object relations, dependency and attachment: A theoretical review of the infant-mother relationship. *Child Development, 40*, 969–1025.
Ainsworth, M., Blehar, M., Waters, E., & Wall, S. (1978). *Patterns of attachment: A psychological study of the Strange situation*. Erlbaum.
Bowlby, J. (1958). The nature of the child's tie to his mother. *The International Journal of Psycho-Analysis, XXXIX*, 1–23.
Bowlby, J. (1959). Separation anxiety. *The International Journal of Psycho-Analysis, XLI*, 1–25.
Bowlby, J. (1960). Grief and mourning in infancy and early childhood. *The Psychoanalytic Student of the Child, VX*, 3–39.
Bowlby, J. (1969). *Attachment and loss. Vol 1: Attachment*. Basic Books.
Bowlby, J. (1973). *Separation: Anxiety and anger*. Basic Books.
Bowlby, J. (1980). *Loss: Sadness and depression*. Basic Books.
Goldstein, J., Solnit, A., Goldstein, S., & Freud, A. (1996). *The best interests of the child: The least detrimental alternative*. The Free Press.
Harlow, H. (1958). The nature of love. *American Psychologist, 13*, 673–685.
Hrdy, S. B. (1999). *Mother nature: A history of mothers, infants, and natural selection*. Pantheon Books.
Main, M., & Solomon, J. (1990). Procedures for identifying infants as disorganized/disoriented during the Ainsworth Strange situation. In M. Greenberg, D. Cicchetti, & E. Cummings (Eds.), *Attachment in the preschool years: Theory, research, and intervention*. The University of Chicago Press.
Masten, A. (2001). Ordinary magic. Resilience processes in development. *American Psychologist, 56*(3), 227–238.
Osofsky, J. (1988). A pioneer in early preventive intervention: A review of *Selected Writings of Selma Fraiberg*. *Merrill-Palmer Quarterly, 34*, 457–460.
Over, H., & Carpenter, M. (2009). Attachment priming improves prosocial behavior in 18-month-olds. *Psychological Science, 20*(10), 1189–1193.
Robertson, J. (1953). Some responses of young children to loss of maternal care. *Nursing Times, 18*, 382–386.
Robertson, J., & Robertson, J. (1989). *Separation and the very young*. Free Association Books.
Stupica, B., Brett, B., Woodhouse, S. S., & Cassidy, J. (2019). Attachment security priming decreases children's physiological response to threat. *Child Development, 90*(4), 1254–1271.
Suomi, S., van der Horst, F., & van der Veer, R. (2008). Rigorous experiments on monkey love: An account of Harry F. Harlow's role in the history of attachment theory. *Integrative Psychological and Behavioral Science, 42*, 354–369.
Warneken, F., & Tomasello, M. (2006). Altruistic helping in human infants and young chimpanzees. *Science, 311*, 1301–1303.

Chapter 2
The IoWA-PCIT Parent Coaching Model

In this chapter, I describe the relationships, research, and theory that inform my attachment-informed parent coaching approach to early-childhood mental health. I provide an overview of the Integration of Working Models of Attachment into Parent–Child Interaction Therapy (IoWA-PCIT) model, the current iteration of how I work with children and families.

Behavioral Parent Coaching

The behavioral parent coaching model that has been most influential in the early-childhood field is the one developed by Connie Hanf (Hanf, 1969). Hanf's parent coaching model for young children with disruptive behavior uses operant conditioning principles to teach parents to use positive attention to shape their child's behavior. Hanf's influence on evidence-based approaches to parent coaching cannot be overestimated. Adaptations of her approach include the following programs: Incredible Years (Webster-Stratton, 1982), Helping the Noncompliant Child (McMahon & Forehand, 2003), and Parent–Child Interaction Therapy (PCIT) (Eyberg & Funderburk, 2011; Eyberg & Matarazzo, 1980; Hembree-Kigin & McNeil, 1995; McNeil & Hembree-Kigin, 2010; Urquiza & McNeil, 1996; Urquiza, Zebell, Timmer, & McGrath, 2012). The research on programs based on Hanf's seemingly simple approach—coach parents to pay attention to child behaviors they want to see more of and to ignore child behaviors they want to see less of—dominates the research on evidence-based approaches to disruptive behavior in young children.

Development of the IoWA-PCIT Parent Coaching Model

My own introduction to the idea of using parent coaching to improve attachment relationships was through the research of Dymphna van den Boom (van den Boom, 1988, 1989, 1994). van den Boom had developed a brief intervention to improve the sensitive responsiveness of mothers to irritable infants. The intervention was grounded in the literature on the development of attachment, but it was also highly individualized—van den Boom coded the interactions of each parent–child dyad and built on the mother's strengths. Specifically, van den Boom's coding of the interaction noted the baby's attachment cues (e.g., positive and negative vocalizations) and the mother's response to the baby's attachment cues. This information was used to coach the mother during interactions with her baby, giving specific feedback about the sensitivity of the mother's responsiveness to the infant and the impact this responsiveness had on the baby. In considering how to address situations where the parent failed to be sensitively responsive to the infant's attachment signals, van den Boom tried to identify where the parent was struggling to respond sensitively to her baby, considering three possible steps: observing the infant's behavior, interpreting the infant's behavior, or determining an appropriate response. I have found this framework extremely helpful in my coaching with families.

In 1996, I learned van den Boom's attachment-informed parent coaching approach (van den Boom, 1988, 1989, 1994), and over the next decade I conducted research focused on the development of irritable infants (Troutman, 2002, 2004a; Troutman, Moran, Arndt, Johnson, & Chmielewski, 2012). But as a clinical psychologist in a department of psychiatry, I rarely received referrals for irritable infants. Instead, as the "attachment person" and the "baby person" in my department, I was sent the youngest children referred (typically preschool-aged) to the department for help. The majority of these children were referred for oppositional and disruptive behavior. Many of these children were in foster care or had been adopted from foster care and had extensive histories of trauma, attachment disruptions, and disruptive behavior. Working with these young patients often felt like a race against time. I knew their disruptive behavior could lead to termination of their foster home or kinship placement and many were on waiting lists for placement in a residential treatment setting. I knew that further disruptions in their attachment relationships and placement in a residential setting were likely to result in more disruptive behavior.

I had begun to apply attachment theory to my clinical work with young children in foster care (Troutman, 2000, 2003, 2004b; Troutman & Cardi, 1998; Troutman, Cardi, & Ryan, 1999; Troutman, Ryan, & Cardi, 2000; Troutman & Wong, 2001). But I knew the important insights gained from research on attachment theory had not yet resulted in interventions that were effectively addressing the significant levels of disruptive behavior and aggression in the young children referred to me. As I scoured the research literature for approaches to addressing disruptive behavior in young children in foster care, I discovered that the approach I had learned in graduate school, behavioral parent coaching, was effective in reducing disruptive behavior in young children in foster care (Fisher, Stollmiller, Gunnar, & Burraston, 2007; Timmer et al., 2006).

In 2006, I headed a project to improve access to evidence-based interventions for child and adolescent mental health problems in Iowa. This project involved bringing trainers to Iowa for a variety of interventions with strong research support. One of these interventions was PCIT (Eyberg & Funderburk, 2011; Eyberg & Matarazzo, 1980; Hembree-Kigin & McNeil, 1995; McNeil & Hembree-Kigin, 2010; Urquiza et al., 2012). At the time that I began disseminating PCIT in Iowa, the only published PCIT protocol was the one published by Hembree-Kigin and McNeil (1995). We were fortunate to have one of the authors of this protocol, Cheryl McNeil, travel to Iowa and Nebraska on several occasions to provide training in the traditional PCIT protocol. (Several different versions of the traditional PCIT protocol have been published since then.) In 2012, Anthony Urquiza and Susan Timmer, researchers whose work changed my perception of the use of behavioral parent coaching for children in foster care, published their PCIT for Traumatized Children protocol (Urquiza et al., 2012).

There were several aspects of PCIT that led me to prefer it to other behavioral parent coaching models. Like van den Boom's (1988, 1989, 1994) attachment-informed interventions for irritable infants, PCIT includes a detailed system for coding the parent's response to the child. Each of the parent's verbalizations to the child is coded, providing a detailed picture of the types of verbalizations the parent directs to the child: positive verbalizations associated with following the child's lead (praising, reflecting, and describing), negative verbalizations (criticizing), and verbalizations associated with directing the child (questions and commands). I liked how this detailed coding provided a framework for giving the parent positive, specific feedback during in vivo coaching. Another aspect of PCIT that I liked was the training model. Training was conducted in small groups with lots of opportunities for therapists to practice the skills and ask questions about potential barriers to implementing the intervention. I saw the potential of PCIT to address the lack of access to services for the group of children I was most concerned about—young children in foster care with disruptive behavior.

I became a PCIT trainer in 2009 and founded the training and research program for PCIT at the University of Iowa. Despite my commitment to making PCIT more accessible, by training community providers in the model, there continued to be some aspects of behavioral parent coaching, in general, and of PCIT, in particular, that I found inconsistent with attachment theory. The aspect I struggled with the most was ignoring the child's distress. In response, over the next few years I developed an integrated approach that incorporated attachment theory research and techniques into PCIT (Troutman, 2015, 2016b, 2016c). This gradual process of developing an attachment-informed parent coaching approach, building on previous work in the field and clinical experience, is described below.

As I coached parents in PCIT, I began making observations about the child's attachment cues and the parent's response to the cues. Rather than viewing crying and distress as indications of "negative attention-seeking behavior," as they were viewed in the traditional PCIT protocols (Eyberg & Funderburk, 2011; Eyberg &

Matarazzo, 1980; Hembree-Kigin & McNeil, 1995; McNeil & Hembree-Kigin, 2010), I viewed them as attachment cues. I had spent so many years immersed in studying attachment theory that this did not seem like an especially radical idea to me. I found that as I made observations about attachment cues to the parent and the parent's response to the cues, parents began to see their children in new ways.

As I struggled to integrate my attachment training into the traditional PCIT protocol, a group of therapists I had trained in the traditional PCIT protocol also became interested in applying attachment theory to their work with parents and children. I began offering workshops on attachment for PCIT therapists, where I shared my ideas about integrating attachment theory into how I delivered PCIT. In these workshops, we discussed the conflicts between attachment theory and behaviorism in regard to parenting young children as well as the overlap between the two approaches. Therapists attending these workshops enthusiastically endorsed incorporating attachment theory into the traditional PCIT protocol. The outcomes I was seeing in my own research, as well as the outcomes the therapists who attended my workshops were seeing, convinced me I was on the right track.

The IoWA-PCIT Model

As noted above, the IoWA-PCIT approach builds on the research on attachment theory and behaviorism and has a huge debt to both. Attachment theory provides the why—the importance of keeping relationships at the center of the intervention—and PCIT provides the how—how to coach parents in strategies for following their child's lead and setting limits that can enhance the parent's relationship with their child and address their child's behavior problems.

In addition to the skills coached in traditional PCIT, in the IoWA-PCIT model, observations of parent–child interactions are used to coach parents in behaviors associated with a more balanced, secure pattern of attachment. The therapist observes the interacting dyad through a one-way mirror and offers help, suggestions, and reinforcement through a communication device in the parent's ear. Emphasis is on positive reinforcement of parents' appropriate behaviors and understanding the parents' lens for responding to their child rather than solely on giving advice for managing their child's behavior.

In dyads with an ambivalent/resistant pattern of attachment, where the dyad is intensely focused on the expression of negative affect, parents are coached to pay more attention to positive affect and savor positive moments. When the dyad is intensely focused on the parent–child relationship, parents are coached to provide support for space and exploration on the part of the child.

In dyads with an avoidant pattern of attachment, where the dyad is focused on the child's failure to ask for help or support, the focus is on helping the parent reinforce the child for asking for help. The focus is also on helping the parent feel comfortable with her child being vulnerable and needing help. In early versions of the protocol, informal observations during behavioral coding were used to determine how to tailor coaching based on the pattern of attachment. In later versions of the protocol, this has been fine-tuned by including a standardized assessment of attachment, administered as part of the pretreatment evaluation for IoWA-PCIT.

In IoWA-PCIT coaching, parenting behaviors associated with secure attachment are reinforced. In dyads where secure attachment is present, I point out to the parent when they respond sensitively to the child's attachment cues and the child's positive response. I also note when the child uses the parent as a secure base for exploration or as a safe haven when they need assistance or comfort. Detailed descriptions of the various attachment patterns and how I tailor the IoWA-PCIT protocol based on these patterns come later in this book.

There are several ways in which research on attachment theory informs the IoWA-PCIT adaptation of traditional PCIT. Most of these differences are seen in process variables—that is, how parents are coached to follow their child's lead and set limits. The adaptations grew from an understanding of factors that promote secure attachment and factors that promote changes from insecure to secure attachment. It is important to approach coaching with an understanding that insecure attachment is adaptive for the child—it enables the child to get their attachment needs met in circumstances where parents have been unable to consistently provide a secure base and/or a safe haven. The parent needs to be better able to meet the child's attachment needs in order for the child to move toward a more secure attachment with the parent. The older the child, the more difficult it will be for them to give up a pattern of attachment that has worked for them and the better they are at hiding their underlying attachment needs.

In IoWA-PCIT coaching, the focus is also on providing parents with the experiences I want them to provide for their child. I'm providing the parent the experience of being in a relationship where they are seen, listened to, and appreciated so that they are able to provide their child with the experience of being seen, listened to, and appreciated. First, since I want the parent to primarily make positive, responsive statements to their child, the majority of my coaching statements are positive and responsive. That is, the vast majority of my coaching statements during Child-Directed Interaction (CDI) (described in Chap. 4) focus on pointing out what the parent is doing right by giving them positive feedback for specific aspects of their parenting. Second, I try to provide the parent with experiences of feeling heard and understood by acknowledging their feelings during interactions, for example, noting that I understand how tough it is when their child ignores them or talks back. Third, I try to provide the parent with experiences of feeling supported during distressing interactions with their child, for example, giving them specific ideas about how to respond to their child's behavior problems and acknowledging the difficulties.

In IoWA-PCIT, parents are taught about the importance of giving attention to their child and the role of child-led play in helping the child develop better emotional regulation. In contrast to more behavioral approaches, in IoWA-PCIT we avoid the term (used in PCIT) "negative attention-seeking behavior" (Eyberg & Funderburk, 2011) to describe the child's motivation for misbehaving. Instead, we concentrate on the power of attention, the inborn need to connect with caregivers that has been repeatedly demonstrated by research on attachment theory.

Using ignoring as a strategy for handling behavior problems is limited to relatively few, carefully defined misbehaviors. Ignoring is not used for crying or other indicators of distress. The concept of differential reinforcement of other behavior (DRO) is emphasized. That is, the focus is on paying attention to alternative behaviors rather than ignoring misbehaviors.

In Parent-Directed Interaction (PDI) (described in Chap. 5), the emphasis is on helping parents remain empathetic and emotionally available to the child at the same time that the parent is teaching the child the very difficult task of following directions. Parents are taught to clearly communicate their expectations to their child in PDI in order to increase compliance and set appropriate limits.

The Integration of Working Models of Attachment into Parent–Child Interaction Therapy (IoWA-PCIT) protocol and handouts are available at https://pcit.lab.uiowa.edu/resources.

Research on IoWA-PCIT

Parenting Factors Associated with Disruptive Behavior

For me, research on the parenting factors associated with disruptive behavior is of more than academic interest. Since I am a therapist, I am interested in mediating factors—that is, parenting factors that we can target in order to decrease disruptive behavior in young children. Thus, one of the first studies I did was to look at the association of attachment and behavioral assessments with parent ratings of disruptive behavior (Troutman, 2017). As anticipated, security of attachment at the initial assessment, as assessed using the Preschool Attachment Classification System (PACS) and Preschool Attachment Rating Scales (PARS) (Cassidy & Marvin, 1992; Moss, Lecompte, & Bureau, 2015), is negatively correlated with parent ratings of disruptive behavior on the Eyberg Child Behavior Inventory (ECBI) (Eyberg & Pincus, 1999). In other words, this research indicates that dyads who are more securely attached have lower ratings of disruptive behavior (Troutman, 2017). In addition, children in dyads who are more securely attached are more compliant with the parent's commands, as assessed using the Dyadic Parent–Child Interaction Coding System (DPICS) (Eyberg, Nelson, Ginn, Bhuiyan, & Boggs, 2013). Thus, one avenue to reducing disruptive behavior and increasing compliance is improving the security of attachment.

The child's rate of compliance at the initial assessment is also negatively correlated with parent ratings of disruptive behavior on the ECBI (Troutman, 2017). That is, children who comply with a greater percentage of their parent's commands have lower ratings of disruptive behavior. Thus, a second avenue to reducing disruptive behavior is increasing compliance by teaching parents to give effective commands, praise compliance, and set limits.

Outcome Studies

My outcome studies of IoWA-PCIT focus on its efficacy with a wide range of families—the types of families referred to me in a Child and Adolescent Psychiatry division. As noted at the beginning of this chapter, I have a particular interest in the efficacy of IoWA-PCIT for young children with disruptive behavior, trauma, and/or attachment disruptions.

In an early study of IoWA-PCIT, I examined whether improvements in disruptive behavior, as assessed by the ECBI, were comparable to the improvements seen in studies of traditional PCIT (Troutman, 2016a, 2016b). I examined the pre- to post-effect sizes using the intent to treat analyses. In other words, I looked at improvement for everyone who started treatment, not just those who completed both phases of treatment. These early results were encouraging. I found statistically significant changes in disruptive behavior with large effect sizes (Cohen's $d > 1$) (Troutman, 2016a, 2016b). These results indicated that my attachment-informed parent coaching approach was at least as robust as the results obtained in traditional PCIT and other behavioral parent training protocols. In a subsequent study, with a larger sample size, I again found statistically significant changes in disruptive behavior and large effect sizes (Cohen's $d > 1$) using the IoWA-PCIT protocol (Troutman, 2016c).

I am especially interested in whether the IoWA-PCIT approach is effective with children with attachment challenges—children who have an insecure attachment relationship with a parent, children who have experienced maltreatment by a parent, and children who have experienced significant disruptions in attachment relationships. In an early study of IoWA-PCIT, I found that security of attachment did not moderate the response to IoWA-PCIT (Troutman, 2016a). In other words, parents in both securely and insecurely attached dyads improve their ability to follow their child's lead during play, and children in both securely and insecurely attached dyads demonstrate significant declines in disruptive behavior. In another early study of IoWA-PCIT, I found significant improvement in disruptive behavior in a sample of adoptees (Troutman, 2016b). The majority of these children had been maltreated by a biological parent prior to adoption and many were referred to me with diagnoses of reactive attachment disorder.

Clinical Experience

As noted above, large effect sizes indicate that the group of children I've treated using IoWA-PCIT demonstrate significant decreases in their behavior problems. However, as their therapist, I know that the path looked different for each child and family. For some dyads, the path was smooth and fast, showing dramatic improvement in a few sessions. For other dyads, the path was rocky and slow, with a few detours along the way, showing slow progress over the course of many sessions. And in the case of a few dyads, we reached a dead end in our work together.

In subsequent chapters, I draw from my clinical experience providing IoWA-PCIT to dyads with different patterns of attachment and parents with different working models of attachment. Knowledge of working models of attachment helps me understand one of the reasons families respond differently to the intervention. By understanding the research on different working models of attachment, I'm better able to understand why some dyads resist change and how to tailor IoWA-PCIT to address their attachment needs and create lasting behavior change.

Training in IoWA-PCIT

Like parenting itself, parent coaching is grounded in relationship and based on procedural memory. Thus, it is useful to receive training and consultation from an experienced IoWA-PCIT trainer. At the time of the publication of this book, almost 700 therapists have been trained in IoWA-PCIT. There are currently 12 IoWA-PCIT trainers providing training in this attachment-informed parent coaching approach through the University of Iowa, University of Nebraska, University of Denver, Plains Area Mental Health Center, Full Circle Therapy Center, Project Harmony, Institute for Therapy and Psychological Solutions, Ampersand Holistic Wellness, Reflect to Connect Psychology, and Restore Therapy & Counseling. Information about receiving training and consultation in IoWA-PCIT is available at https://pcit.lab.uiowa.edu/.

The Bottom Line

The IoWA-PCIT protocol for coaching parents during interactions with their child is a highly effective method of improving the child–parent relationship and addressing the child's behavior problems. The reason the IoWA-PCIT approach is so effective is that it builds on decades of research based on attachment theory and behaviorism and the clinical wisdom of therapists I have learned from over the years.

References

Cassidy, J., & Marvin, R. (1992). *Attachment organization in preschool children: Procedures and coding manual*. University of Virginia.

Eyberg, S., & Funderburk, B. (2011). *Parent-child interaction therapy protocol*. PCIT International, Inc..

Eyberg, S., & Matarazzo, R. (1980). Training parents as therapists: A comparison between individual parent-child interaction training and parent group didactic training. *Journal of Clinical Psychology, 36*, 492–499.

References

Eyberg, S., & Pincus, D. (1999). *Eyberg child behavior inventory and sutter-eyberg student behavior inventory – revised.* Psychological Assessment Resources.

Eyberg, S., Nelson, M., Ginn, N., Bhuiyan, N., & Boggs, S. (2013). *Dyadic Parent-Child Interaction Coding System (DPICS): Comprehensive manual for research and training.* PCIT International, Inc..

Fisher, P., Stollmiller, M., Gunnar, M., & Burraston, B. (2007). Effects of a therapeutic intervention for foster preschoolers on diurnal cortisol activity. *Psychoneuroendocrinology, 32,* 892–905.

Hanf, C. (1969). *A two-stage program for modifying maternal controlling during mother-child (M-C) interaction.* Paper presented at the Western Psychological Association.

Hembree-Kigin, T., & McNeil, C. (1995). *Parent-child interaction therapy.* Plenum Press.

McMahon, R., & Forehand, R. (2003). *Helping the noncompliant child* (2nd ed.). Guilford.

McNeil, C., & Hembree-Kigin, T. (2010). *Parent-child interaction therapy* (2nd ed.). Springer.

Moss, E., Lecompte, V., & Bureau, J. (2015). *Preschool and early school-age attachment rating scales (PARS).* University of Quebec at Montreal.

Timmer, S., Urquiza, A., Herschell, A., McGrath, J., Zebell, N., Porter, A., & Vargas, E. (2006). Parent-child interaction therapy: Application of an empirically supported treatment to maltreated children in foster care. *Child Welfare: Journal of Policy, Practice, and Program, 85*(6), 919–939.

Troutman, B. (2000). *Using attachment theory to guide clinical work with young children in foster care.* Paper presented at the Department of Psychology Clinical Psychology Seminar, University of Iowa.

Troutman, B. (2002). *Assessment of infant irritability in early infancy.* Paper presented at the Proceedings of the World Assocation for Infant Mental Health 8th World Congress.

Troutman, B. (2003). *Meeting the needs of young children in foster care: Evidence-based models of assessment and intervention.* Paper presented at the The Fourth Annual Ohio Association for Infant Mental Health (OAIMH) Conference. Back from the Edge: Relationship-based interventions.

Troutman, B. (2004a). *Assessing infants of mothers who took SSRIs during pregnancy.* Paper presented at the Proceedings of the Marce Society International Biennial Scientific Meeting.

Troutman, B. (2004b). *Meeting the development and mental health needs of young children in foster care.* Paper presented at the Advancing public health: Meeting the challenge, 2004 Public Health Conference.

Troutman, B. (2015). *Integrating behaviorism and attachment theory in parent coaching.* Springer.

Troutman, B. (2016a). Does security of attachment moderate response to parent-child intervention for disruptive behavior? In K. Alvarez (Ed.), *Parent-child interactions and relationships: Perceptions, practice and developmental outcomes* (pp. 45–60). Nova Publishers.

Troutman, B. (2016b). Integrated behaviorism and attachment theory approach to reducing disruptive behavior in young adoptees. In K. Alvarez (Ed.), *Parent-child interactions and relationships: Perceptions, practices, and developmental outcomes* (pp. 61–74). Nova Publishers.

Troutman, B. (2016c). *Integrating behaviorism and attachment theory in addressing disruptive behavior.* Paper presented at the 63rd Annual Meeting of the American Academy of Child & Adolescent Psychiatry.

Troutman, B. (2017). *Using pre-treatment interaction assessments to guide coching.* Paper presented at the 2017 PCIT International Convention, Traverse City.

Troutman, B., & Cardi, M. (1998). *Helping young children in foster care develop healthy attachments.* Paper presented at the Proceedings of the Zero to Three 13th National Training Institute.

Troutman, B., & Wong, M. (2001). *Effects of neglect on developmental functioning.* Paper presented at the Proceedings of the Zero to Three 16th National Training Institute.

Troutman, B., Cardi, M., & Ryan, S. (1999). Infants placed in out-of-home care: Implications for attachment. *The Source, 9*(3), 12–15.

Troutman, B., Ryan, S., & Cardi, M. (2000). The effects of foster care placement on young children's mental health. *Protecting Children, 16*(1), 30–34.

Troutman, B., Moran, T. E., Arndt, S., Johnson, R. F., & Chmielewski, M. (2012). Development of parenting self-efficacy in mothers of infants with high negative emotionality. *Infant Ment Health J, 33*(1). https://doi.org/10.1002/imhj.20332

Urquiza, A., & McNeil, C. (1996). Parent-child interaction therapy: An intensive dyadic intervention for physically abusive families. *Child Maltreatment, 1*(2), 134–144.

Urquiza, A., Zebell, N., Timmer, S., & McGrath, J. (2012). *Course of Treatment Manual for PCIT-TC*. University of California Davis.

van den Boom, D. (1988). *Neonatal irritability and the development of attachment: Observation and intervention*. Dissertation, University of Leiden.

van den Boom, D. (1989). Neonatal irritability and the development of attachment. In G. Kohnstamm, J. Bates, & M. Rothbart (Eds.), *Temperament in Childhood*. John Wiley & Sons.

van den Boom, D. (1994). The influence of temperament and mothering on attachment and exploration: An experimental manipulation of sensitive responsiveness among lower-class mothers with irritable infants. *Child Development, 65*, 1457–1477.

Webster-Stratton, C. (1982). Teaching mothers through videotape modeling to change their children's behavior. *Journal of Pediatric Psychology, 7*(3), 279–294.

Chapter 3
How to Complete an Attachment-Informed Early-Childhood Mental Health Assessment

In this chapter, I describe how to keep the focus on relationships when completing an assessment of a young child's mental health problems. I describe how to conduct an intake and initial assessment for Integration of Working Models of Attachment into Parent–Child Interaction Therapy (IoWA-PCIT) that attends to the relationship the therapist is developing with the parent and the child. I also describe how to conduct observational assessments that help us understand early-childhood mental health problems within the context of attachment relationships. Specifically, I discuss how to conduct an attachment assessment based on the Preschool Strange Situation Procedure and a behavioral assessment based on the Dyadic Parent–Child Interaction Coding System (DPICS). I discuss how the assessment period is a critical period for forming a therapeutic alliance with parents and children and describe how to foster these relationships during the assessment.

Understanding Problems in a Relationship Context

Our mental health system is based on the idea that mental health problems reside in the individual. However, infant and early-childhood mental health assessments place an emphasis on assessing the relationship between the parent and child. Unfortunately, given the bias of our mental health system, some therapists view the problem as residing in the parent or feel they need to evaluate which individual the problem resides in, the parent or the child.

Conducting an infant and early-childhood mental health assessment requires a fundamental shift in how we view mental health. It means starting with the premise that "a baby alone does not exist" (Winnicott, 1987). In other words, when we conduct an infant and early-childhood mental health assessment, we start with an understanding of the dependence of infants and young children on their relationship with their parents. In the IoWA-PCIT pretreatment mental health assessment, we evaluate young children within a relational context because whatever the etiology of the problems the child is experiencing, those difficulties will be expressed within the relationship with their parents.

Goals of Attachment-Informed Assessment

The goals when completing an attachment-informed assessment of a young child referred for mental health concerns are threefold: (1) forming a therapeutic alliance with the parents and child, (2) understanding the parent's concerns about the child within the context of their views of relationships, and (3) conducting observational assessments that help us understand the child's emotional and behavioral problems within the context of their most important relationships. The observational assessments utilized in the pretreatment assessment for IoWA-PCIT examine the quality of the child–parent attachment relationships, the parent's positive and negative verbalizations to the child during child-led play, and the child's compliance with the parent's commands during parent-led play and cleanup.

Careful assessment is an important part of laying the groundwork for effective parent coaching. However, as Ainsworth stated when talking about developing a system for classifying patterns of attachment, "Preoccupation with measurement may lead one to forget that this is a tool and not an end in itself" (Ainsworth, Blehar, Waters, & Wall, 1978). This is an important rule to keep in mind during the assessment: Our observations of parent–child interactions are a tool for providing effective intervention, not the end goal.

What Parents of Infants and Young Children Need from Therapists

It's important to think about what parents of infants and young children need from us, as we conduct an infant or early-childhood mental health assessment. This assessment is a critical time in forming a therapeutic alliance between the therapist and the parent. Therefore, it's helpful to begin considering the parent's needs as early as the initial assessment.

Considering the parent's attachment needs and the vulnerable position of a parent reaching out to a therapist for help starts with our first encounter with the parent. The goal is to treat the parent as the expert on their particular child while presenting ourselves as the experts in supporting them and their child in achieving their goals. As I listen to the parent's concerns, I am thinking about how to place these concerns within the context of their community, their current stressors, and their family. For example, having a 3-year-old with disruptive behavior who is at risk of being kicked out of their childcare setting may put considerable stress on a family if it interferes with the parent's ability to work.

Just as young children need to be seen and heard, parents of young children need to have their efforts and struggles acknowledged during the assessment. I will never forget a conversation I had with the mother of an infant following a talk on attachment. She said that she thought people forget how difficult it is to care for an infant. I realized that my well-intentioned talk on the attachment needs of infants had failed to acknowledge the attachment needs of new parents—for example, how difficult it is to meet the attachment needs of an infant while sleep-deprived.

Like sensitively responsive parents, sensitive therapists must recognize what parents want while providing what they need. It sometimes seems like what parents want is easy answers, or, better yet, to be told that they can continue handling situations the way they are currently handling them and get a different outcome. We can also acknowledge the parent's need to be told this, even if we aren't able to meet it. Most importantly, we need to acknowledge the parent's positive intention even if their interactions with their child do not appear consistent with this intention.

It can be challenging to get parents to change their ways of interacting with their child. At the initial assessment, I am laying the groundwork for our work together as I listen to the parent's concerns. I am thinking about what this parent will need from me in order to change their current way of interacting with their child. There is no way of getting around the fact that our relationship with the parent is critical to our success as early-childhood interventionists. The parent needs the type of relationship we want them to provide for their child—a relationship where it is safe to be vulnerable and explore new ways of being with their child. In the words of Philip Bromberg, "New words about the self can be tasted pleasurably only in the safety of a relational context that provides a sense of security and continuity" (Bromberg, 2011a).

Let's be honest: Even in the context of a warm and supportive relationship, learning that you have contributed to your child's problems, however inadvertently, may not always be tasted pleasurably. But these new words are unlikely to be tasted at all without establishing a secure therapeutic relationship with the parent.

Parent's Working Models of Attachment

I begin to consider the parent's internal working models of attachment during assessment by listening closely to how they talk to their child and to me. Understanding a parent's working model of attachment can help me understand why parents might resist changing their patterns of interactions with their child. It also provides me with information that helps me tailor the parent coaching.

Considering the parent's working model of attachment helps me have empathy for the parent and understand their perceptions, especially when their working model of attachment leads them to communicate in ways that make parent coaching more challenging for me as the therapist. More details on recognizing and working with parents with different working models of attachment are provided in Chaps. 8, 10, 12, and 14.

What I used to view as a challenge, translating parenting strategies for parents with different working models of attachment, I now see as an opportunity. It is like a two-for-one special. By helping the parent find new, more secure ways of interacting with me and their child, I am having a positive impact on both the parent and the child. As I describe in Chap. 17, this is actually more like a three-for-one special: It turns out that translating relationship concepts for parents with different working models of attachment has been an opportunity for my growth as well.

Jeree Pawl recommends applying what she calls the platinum rule to working with parents of young children: "Do unto others as you would have others do unto others" (Lieberman & Van Horn, 2008). Or, as a participant in one of my workshops said, it's like parenting the parent so that they can parent the child. Luckily, we have the biological predisposition for caregiving and attachment on our side. Parents' investment in their young children means they are willing to make changes for the sake of their children. Making these changes sometimes feels like going against everything the parent knows to be true, a very scary proposition for them. It is only for the sake of their child and because of the positive effect they see changes having on their child, that parents are willing to make this leap into the unknown. We cannot make this leap for them. But we can provide a secure base for their exploration and a safe haven when the going gets tough.

Infants and young children adapt their strategies for getting their attachment needs met to a particular caregiver. Thus, they can have different patterns of attachment with different parents.

Adults develop an internal working model of attachment based on their own early attachment experiences. This working model—that is, the blueprint for being in relationships the parent brings to all relationships—informs their adult attachment relationships. As therapists, we have at least two sources of information regarding the parent's internal working model of attachment. The first source is observations of how the parent interacts with the child during sessions. The second source is the language the parent uses to communicate their needs to us. The research on internal working models of attachment is based on adults' use of language to communicate with an interviewer about their history. This area of research began with the development of the Adult Attachment Interview (AAI) (George, Kaplan, & Main, 1984; Main, 2000a, 2000b). Learning to code the AAI and conducting research on adult attachment (Caspers , Paradiso, Yucuis, Troutman, Arndt, & Philibert, 2009; Caspers, Cadoret, Langbehn, Yucuis, & Troutman, 2005; Caspers, Yucuis, Troutman, Arndt, & Langbehn, 2007; Caspers, Yucuis, Troutman, & Spinks, 2006) fundamentally changed the way I listened to parents in therapy.

The aspect of the AAI I find most intriguing is that it is *how* parents tell the story of their childhood—not the content—that reveals their internal working model (Mary Main and her colleagues refer to this as state of mind) (George et al., 1984; Main, 2000a, 2000b). Basically, parents of infants with secure infant–parent attachment strategies are good storytellers. In response to a series of questions about their childhood experiences, they communicate with the interviewer in a way that is clear, concise, and consistent, and takes the perspective of the interviewer into account. When they answer the questions about their childhood, their answers are fresh, as though they are thinking about the questions and reflecting on their answers. When they describe difficult experiences during their childhood, experiences where their parents had failed to meet their attachment needs, they place these experiences in context and are forgiving of their parents' failures to meet their needs.

In understanding how to tailor parent coaching to meet the parent's attachment needs, I have found two bodies of research especially helpful: research on the relationship between the parent's internal working model of attachment and their child's pattern of attachment (Main, 2000a, 2000b; H. Steele & Steele, 2005, 2008; M. Steele, Hodges, Kaniuk, Steele, Hillman, & Asquith 2008; van Ijzendoorn, 1995) and research on how working models of attachment influence a patient's relationship with their therapist (Caspers et al., 2006; Dozier, 1990, 2001; Dozier, Cue, & Barnett, 1994; Korfmacher, Adam, Ogawa, & Egeland, 1997; Miller-Bottome, Talia, Eubanks, Safran, & Muran, 2019; Miller-Bottome, Talia, Safran, & Muran, 2017; Talia, Daniel, Miller-Bottome, Brambilla, Miccoli, Safran, & Lingiardi.et al., 2014; Talia, Miller-Bottome, & Daniel, 2015). We are in a unique role when we are doing therapeutic work with parents and their young children—our focus is on the relationship. However, in order to focus on the relationship, we need to attend to both the child's and the parent's attachment needs.

My goal is to involve each primary caregiver in parent coaching. This means I have to translate the approach for individuals with different, and sometimes competing, working models of attachment. Gathering clues about the parents' working models of attachment begins at this initial assessment but continues throughout our work with the family.

Initial Intake

At the initial intake, I let the parents know I am interested in their perspective on their child's problems. I find it important to figure out a way to spend time talking with the parent without the child present so the parent can speak freely about their concerns.

When did they first become concerned about their child? What do they think has led to the problems? What have they done to address the problems? Who have they talked with about their child's problems (either voluntarily because they sought help or involuntarily because someone suggested they needed to "do something" about their child's behavior problems)? I let the parents know that I have expertise in working with other families where the child has behavior problems and am looking forward to using this expertise to tailor intervention to their family. At this session, I typically have the parent complete an Eyberg Child Behavior Inventory (ECBI) (Eyberg & Pincus, 1999), a brief assessment of disruptive behavior as well as other assessments that may be indicated by presenting problems.

Of course, I am also thinking about the child's attachment needs in these initial encounters and about forming a relationship with the child. But this seems to be the easiest part of the assessment process. Children seem to intuitively understand that the therapist is trying to help them and their parent. There are also a number of ways we can enhance our therapeutic alliance with the child. First, I am transparent with children about the reasons for the evaluation. I try to sum up the referral question in a couple of sentences such as "You are coming here with your parents to see me because they are worried about how you have been getting in a lot of trouble at home. I am the kind of doctor who helps children and parents get along better. I will be watching you and your parents from behind that mirror so I can get some ideas about how to help you." My understanding of the developmental needs of young children and my ability to engage in child-led play also facilitate the establishment of a therapeutic alliance with the child. In other words, for the brief periods of time I spend interacting with the child, I am using the child-led play skills described in Chap. 4.

The long-term goal is to help the parent better meet the child's attachment needs. However, if I jump too quickly to trying to get the parent to interact differently with their child, without understanding the parent's needs, my work with the parent–child dyad will not truly be attachment-informed.

Pretreatment Assessment for IoWA-PCIT

At the pretreatment assessment for IoWA-PCIT, most of my time is spent observing child–parent interactions from behind a one-way mirror or through a video monitor. It is probably a truism to say that relationships are more complex than our ability to analyze relationships. However, by using standardized assessments and standardized ways of analyzing dyadic interactions, I have a lens that helps me identify strengths and struggles from both an attachment and social learning perspective. I will gain a richer understanding of the family as treatment continues, but this initial understanding of the family's strengths and struggles gives me a road map to guide my coaching.

I use a communication device placed in the parent's ear to give them instructions about each part of the observation. I try to observe the child with each parent prior to beginning treatment. The observations are of a dyad—for example, child–mother dyad and child–father dyad. If more than one child from a family is referred for treatment, I try to do an observation of each child with at least one parent.

Attachment Assessment (Preschool Strange Situation Procedure)

The first set of observations helps me understand the child's strategy for getting their attachment needs met with each parent. This is a 25-minute observation of the child's reactions to a series of brief (5-minute) separations and reunions. The observation strategy is based on the Strange Situation Procedure used in research on attachment (Ainsworth et al., 1978; Cassidy & Marvin, 1992; Main & Solomon, 1990; Moss, Cyr, & Dubois-Comtois, 2004; Moss, Lecompte, & Bureau, 2015). (The Preschool Strange Situation Procedure is often referred to as the separation–reunion procedure for preschool-aged children in the research literature in order to differentiate it from the Strange Situation Procedure used with infants.)

In subsequent chapters, I will go into more detail about how this attachment assessment provides information about how to tailor parent coaching. As I watch separations and reunions between young children and their parents, I'm reminded of the power of early relationships, regardless of the pattern of attachment or the extent of the struggles in the dyad. This opportunity to be reminded that we are born for relationships is one of the perks of my work.

Behavioral Assessment (Dyadic Parent–Child Interaction Coding System)

The second set of observations gives me a window into how the parent communicates with the child and the child's compliance with parent directives. Parent verbalizations and child compliance are coded during three different brief (5 minute) situations. The coding used for these observations is based on the Dyadic Parent–Child Interaction Coding System (DPICS) (Eyberg, Nelson, Ginn, Bhuiyan, & Boggs, 2013) used in research on behavioral parent coaching interventions based on social learning theory. The first of these situations involves a 5-minute observation where the parent is told to let the child choose an activity and play along with the child (child-led play). Coding the parent's verbalizations to the child during this situation serves as a proxy for understanding what aspects of the child's behavior the parent attends to—for example, whether the parent is focused on criticizing the child's behavior or on praising the child's behavior. This observation also yields two summary variables that are important to understanding the parent's approach to interactions during a low-stress situation—positive following (the number of times the parent praises the child, describes the child's behavior, or reflects what the child said) and negative leading (the number of times the parent criticizes the child, tells the child what to do, or asks a question).

DPICS coding also provides information about the child's compliance with the parent's commands during the situation where the parent is told to choose the activity and keep the child playing with the parent according to the parent's rules (parent-led play) and during the situation where the parent is told to have the child clean up the toys by themselves (cleanup).

One of the most striking aspects of this part of the evaluation is the number of commands parents give during these 5 minutes. As someone who doesn't like to be told what to do, I identify with the child and find it jarring to think about being given a command approximately every 10 seconds (I find parents give an average of 55 commands during the 10 minutes of parent-led play and cleanup at the initial evaluation for IoWA-PCIT). When viewed from the child's perspective, being able to follow this number of commands seems like an impossible task.

When watching these interactions, it is easy to wonder why parents give so many commands when it is so obviously frustrating for their child. It's important to keep in mind that the parent is seeking services because of the conflictual relationship with their child and their child's oppositional behavior. From the parent's perspective, they need to give a lot of commands because their experience is their child is unlikely to comply. It appears their strategy is to throw out a lot of commands in hope some of them will eventually stick.

Getting an initial assessment is important, but I also keep in mind that establishing a strong therapeutic relationship with the parent and child is paramount. For example, if the child becomes extremely distressed during the separation from the parent and is fearful about a second separation, there is no need to do a second separation.

If the child becomes aggressive during the initial assessment, I enter the room with a flourish to distract them and disrupt the aggression. Making a dramatic entrance serves as a distraction for both the parent and the child and diffuses the tension. One of the important things to keep in mind as an attachment-informed therapist is the need to gauge our interventions to what the dyad is ready to tolerate. It is certainly tempting to rush in during an assessment and start giving advice about how to handle behavior. However, giving advice at this point may undermine the therapeutic relationship with both the child and the parent. Instead, the focus is on interrupting the aggression and setting the stage for our work together.

Clues to Parent's Working Model of Attachment

I don't administer a standardized assessment of working model of attachment to parents. Instead, I rely on several clues to their working model that are informed by the research on attachment theory: (1) how the parent interacts with the child; (2) the parent's perceptions of the child—especially the gap between my observations of interactions and the parent's perceptions; (3) how the parent communicates with me; and (4) my countertransference reaction to the parent. These clues, described in more detail in Chaps. 8, 10, 12, and 14, are based on research on the Adult Attachment Interview (AAI), including research on how individuals with different working models of attachment communicate with therapists (Caspers et al., 2005; Caspers et al., 2006; Caspers et al., 2007; Caspers et al., 2009; Dozier, 1990; Dozier et al., 1994; George et al., 1984; Main, 2000a, 2000b; Miller-Bottome et al., 2017; Miller-Bottome et al., 2019; Talia et al., 2014; Talia et al., 2015). I also draw on my clinical experience, including the pitfalls I have fallen into with parents with different types of working models of attachment.

Just as our goal is to understand how the child's working model of attachment leads them to behave in certain ways with the parent, our goal is to understand how the parent's working model of attachment leads them to behave in certain ways with us and with their child. Nobody sets out to be a bad parent—especially not a parent who is seeking help. Two of the questions I hope to begin answering by the end of the initial assessment are "Why does the parent think the child behaves the way they do?" and "What does this tell me about the parent's view of relationships?"

I find the Adult Attachment Interview's (AAI) (George et al., 1984; Main, 2000b) distinction between showing and telling useful in conceptualizing the initial evaluation. That is, what the parent *showed* me about their relationship with the child—that is, what I observed happening between them and the child—and what the parent *told* me about their relationship or the child's behavior. None of us is able to see ourselves as others see us, but the larger the discrepancy between what parents show us and what they tell us, the more important it will be to keep the parent's model of attachment in mind during our work together.

A typical example of a discrepancy between the parent's perceptions and my observations of the child's behavior is that children referred for disruptive behavior are typically better behaved than expected. Another example is when a parent tells me their child is unable to separate from them for even a brief period of time without becoming intensely distressed. Yet, the child exhibits minimal distress during the brief separation that occurs as part of the assessment.

As we reflect on the discrepancy between our perceptions of the child and the parent's perceptions, it is important to hold our ideas lightly. After all, the parent has an extensive history of observing the child prior to the evaluation. I think of these discrepancies as informing us about the child's potential—their potential to engage in prosocial behavior or manage anxiety about a brief separation in certain circumstances.

The discrepancies I am especially interested in are the discrepancies between parents' view of their parenting and my observations of their interactions with their child. A typical example is parents who describe themselves as being knowledgeable about the importance of praise and positive attention and believe they frequently give their child positive attention but rarely praise their child's positive behavior during the initial evaluation. There are numerous possible reasons for this discrepancy. The parent may have a different definition of positive behavior than I do—that is, they may have much higher standards for what they consider appropriate behavior. Another possibility is that the parent has a different definition of positive attention—that is, while we are coding verbal attention (praise, reflection, and behavior description) to the child's behavior, the parent may consider a brief look or smile to be sufficient acknowledgment. Some parents have their own mental health problems or attachment trauma that interferes with their ability to see their child's positive behavior when they interact with the child—instead, they "see" someone from their past who is not deserving of positive attention.

Moving forward, it is important to stay curious about these discrepancies and provide a space where parents have an opportunity to notice and wonder about these discrepancies themselves. There is something about the shared space provided when we are observing the same interaction during parent coaching (described in detail in subsequent chapters) that often allows them to do this. At the initial evaluation, our goal is to use observations of potential discrepancies to have some ideas about the blind spots that keep the parents from being the kind of parents they want to be. One question I frequently get asked by therapists is why I don't just tell parents about the potential blind spots I identify during the initial evaluation. It's a reasonable question. My experience is that working models of attachment serve as defenses that protect people from seeing things about themselves they are not yet ready to see. There are likely a few sturdy souls who could recognize that they aren't who they think they are in relationships but, for most people, it is a kick in the gut to hear feedback about the discrepancy between who they *tell* us they are in relationship and what they *show* us about who they are in relationship. It takes an established therapeutic relationship where they feel accepted and valued to be able to look at these discrepancies.

Much has been written about parents' reflective functioning, how it relates to parenting, and how it relates to their ability to make use of therapy (Slade, 2005). One aspect of reflective functioning is the ability to notice discrepancies between what we show and what we tell. Noticing this discrepancy can be the first step to narrowing the discrepancy. One of the ways this happens is through the feedback we give each week after we observe and give feedback at the beginning of the session. Parents will begin to realize that they may not be as good at noticing their child's positive behavior as they thought.

Although noticing the discrepancy and reflecting on it is an important path to changing the pattern of interaction, I don't think it's the only way. Some parents are able to show up in their relationship with their child in a way that is more consistent with what they tell us, once they begin IoWA-PCIT, even without having discrepancies pointed out. Philip Bromberg describes a similar phenomenon in his work with patients by stating that "change precedes insight" (Bromberg, 2011b). In other words, sometimes you need to act differently in relationship before you can have insight into your contribution to the pattern of interaction. At this initial evaluation, we need to notice these discrepancies and begin building a therapeutic relationship with the parent that provides a safe space for them to find new ways of interacting with their child.

The statements I make to parents and children at the end of the initial evaluation pave the way for our work together—the tough work of beginning to make changes in their interactions. I describe the strengths I see in their relationship and in them as individuals and share my sense of hope that we will be able to build on those strengths.

The Bottom Line

When completing an attachment-informed early-childhood mental health assessment, the crucial role of relationships in healing and development is kept at the forefront. First, we must keep in mind the importance of establishing a therapeutic relationship with the parent and child that honors what each contributes to the current struggles as well as the potential for growth and improvement in their interactions. During the assessment, we are forming a relationship with the parent that is based, at least in part, on the parent's working model of attachment—the same model that informs their relationship with their child. Second, we conduct the evaluation in such a way that the focus is on the context in which the problems occur—parent–child interactions. We conduct an observational assessment of their relationship that focuses on the ways in which they navigate the balance between attachment and exploration in their relationship. We also conduct an observational assessment of their relationship that focuses on the parent's verbal communication with the child and the child's compliance with the parent's commands.

References

Ainsworth, M., Blehar, M., Waters, E., & Wall, S. (1978). *Patterns of attachment: A psychological study of the strange situation*. Erlbaum.

Bromberg, P. (2011a). *Awakening the dreamer*. Taylor & Francis.

Bromberg, P. (2011b). *The shadow of the Tsunami and the growth of the relational mind*. Taylor & Francis Group, LLC.

Caspers, K. M., Cadoret, R. J., Langbehn, D., Yucuis, R., & Troutman, B. (2005). Contributions of attachment style and perceived social support to lifetime use of illicit substances. *Addictive Behaviors, 30*(5), 1007–1011.

Caspers, K. M., Yucuis, R., Troutman, B., & Spinks, R. (2006). Attachment as an organizer of behavior: Implications for substance abuse problems and willingness to seek treatment. *Substance Abuse Treatment, Prevention, and Policy, 1*.

Caspers, K. M., Yucuis, R., Troutman, B., Arndt, S., & Langbehn, D. (2007). A sibling adoption study of adult attachment: The influence of shared environment on attachment state of mind. *Attachment & Human Development, 9*(4), 375–391.

Caspers, K. M., Paradiso, S., Yucuis, R., Troutman, B., Arndt, S., & Philibert, R. (2009). Association between the serotonin transporter promoter polymorphism (5-HTTLPR) and adult unresolved attachment. *Development Psychology, 45*(1), 64–76.

Cassidy, J., & Marvin, R. (1992). *Attachment organization in preschool children: Procedures and coding manual*. University of Virginia.

Dozier, M. (1990). Attachment organization and treatment use for adults with serious psychopathological disorders. *Development and Psychopathology, 2*, 47–60.

Dozier, M. (2001). The challenge of treatment for clients with dismissing state of mind. *Attachment & Human Development, 3*(1), 62–76.

Dozier, M., Cue, K., & Barnett, L. (1994). Clinicians as caregivers: Role of attachment organization in treatment. *Journal of Consulting and Clinical Psychology, 62*(4).

Eyberg, S., & Pincus, D. (1999). *Eyberg child behavior inventory and sutter-eyberg student behavior inventory – revised*. Psychological Assessment Resources.

Eyberg, S., Nelson, M., Ginn, N., Bhuiyan, N., & Boggs, S. (2013). *Dyadic Parent-Child Interaction Coding System (DPICS): Comprehensive manual for research and training*. PCIT International, Inc..

George, C., Kaplan, N., & Main, M. (1984). *Adult attachment interview*. University of California.

Korfmacher, J., Adam, E., Ogawa, J., & Egeland, B. (1997). Adult attachment: Implications for the therapeutic process in a home visitation intervention. *Applied Developmental Science, 1*(1), 43–52.

Lieberman, A., & Van Horn, P. (2008). *Psychotherapy with infants and young children: Repairing the effects of stress and trauma on early attachment*. The Guilford Press.

Main, M. (2000a). Disorganized infant, child, and adult attachment: Collapse in behavioral and attentional strategies. *Journal of the American Psychoanalytic Association, 48*.

Main, M. (2000b). The organized categories of infant, child, and adult attachment: Flexible vs. inflexible attention under attachment-related stress. *Journal of the American Psychoanalytic Association, 48*.

Main, M., & Solomon, J. (1990). Procedures for identifying infants as disorganized/disoriented during the Ainsworth Strange situation. In M. Greenberg, D. Cicchetti, & E. Cummings (Eds.), *Attachment in the preschool years: Theory, research, and intervention*. The University of Chicago Press.

Miller-Bottome, M., Talia, A., Safran, J., & Muran, J. (2017). Resolving alliance ruptures from an attachment-informed perspective. *Psychoanalytic Psychology*.

Miller-Bottome, M., Talia, A., Eubanks, C., Safran, J., & Muran, J. (2019). Secure in-session attachment predicts rupture resolution: Negotiating a secure base. *Psychoanalytic Psychology, 36*(2), 132–138.

Moss, E., Cyr, C., & Dubois-Comtois, K. (2004). Attachment at early school age and developmental risk: Examining family contexts and behavior problems of controlling-caregiving, controlling-punitive, and behaviorally disorganized children. *Developmental Psychology, 40*(4), 519–532.

Moss, E., Lecompte, V., & Bureau, J. (2015). *Preschool and early school-age attachment rating scales (PARS)*. University of Quebec at Montreal.

Slade, A. (2005). Parental reflective functioning: An introduction. *Attachment & Human Development, 7*(3), 269–281.

Steele, H., & Steele, M. (2005). Understanding and resolving emotional conflict: The London parent-child project. In K. Grossman, K. Grossman, & E. Waters (Eds.), *Attachment from infancy to adulthood: The major longitudinal studies*. The Guilford Press.

Steele, H., & Steele, M. (2008). *Clinical applications of the adult attachment interview*. The Guilford Press.

Steele, M., Hodges, J., Kaniuk, J., Steele, H., Hillman, S., & Asquith, K. (2008). Forecasting outcomes in previously maltreated children: The use of the AAI in a longitudinal adoption study. In H. Steele & M. Steele (Eds.), *Clinical applications of the adult attachment interview*. The Guilford Press.

Talia, A., Daniel, S., Miller-Bottome, M., Brambilla, D., Miccoli, D., Safran, J., & Lingiardi, V. (2014). AAI predicts patients' in-session interpersonal behavior and discourse: A "move to the level of the relation" for attachment-informed psychotherapy research. *Attachment & Human Development, 16*(2), 192–209.

Talia, A., Miller-Bottome, M., & Daniel, S. (2015). Assessing attachment in psychotherapy: Validation study of the patient attachment coding system. *Clinical Psychology & Psychotherapy, 24*, 149–161.

van Ijzendoorn, M. (1995). Adult attachment representations, parental responsiveness, and infant attachment: A meta-analysis on the predictive validity of the adult attachment interview. *Psychological Bulletin, 117*(3), 387–403.

Winnicott, D. W. (1987). *Babies and their mothers*. Addison-Wesley Publishing Company, Inc.

Chapter 4
How to Coach Parents to Follow Their Child's Lead in Play

In this chapter, I describe how to coach parents to follow their child's lead during play—the core foundation of improving the child–parent relationship and the child's social-emotional functioning. I describe how to present the Child-Directed Interaction (CDI) skills to the parent during an engage and teach session and how to coach the parent to follow their child's lead during play.

Born to Play

Play scholar Peter Gray argues that we are born to play (Gray, 2009, 2011, 2013). Like attachment, play is part of our evolutionary heritage. According to Gray, there are five characteristics of play (Gray, 2009). First, play is an activity the individual chooses and directs. In other words, it's not truly playful if someone is telling you how to play. I sometimes smile to myself when parents or therapists ask how they will get a child to play. It is almost like asking how you will get a child to breathe. As soon as a child enters a room, they will begin playing. They may not always choose to play with the toys I have selected for them, instead playing with the light switch, the container the toys were in, or a piece of lint on the floor. But I assure you they will choose to play given the opportunity.

Second, Gray argues that play is intrinsically motivated. In other words, children play because they want to and find it enjoyable—not because it is required. Third, although children have the freedom to play or not to play, they must follow certain rules to be included in play with others. For example, in play fighting it is important to not really hurt the other person. Gray notes that because children must learn to follow rules in order to play with others, "children learn that inhibiting their impulses is not only necessary but is, ultimately, a source of pleasure" (Gray, 2013).

The fourth feature of play identified by Gray is that it is imaginative. This creative aspect of play provides the child with the opportunity of learning new ways of being in the world. Children can literally play with possibilities. Fifth, Gray notes the frame of mind during play is alert but relatively unstressed. Sometimes, we forget just how stressful the demands of childhood can be—especially for a child who struggles with self-regulation and compliance. Play is a time when children can relax and enjoy themselves.

Benefits of Child-Led Play with a Parent

Child-led play with a parent provides an opportunity for the child to explore new ways of being in relationship and, with the parents' scaffolding, engage in better behavior and regulation than they do when they are stressed. In addition, when parents spend time doing child-led play with their child, they are physically near the child in a low-demand situation, making it easier for the parent to recognize and respond to the child's attachment signals.

Research on play therapy indicates it is effective for a wide variety of emotional and behavioral problems, and the most effective play therapy approaches are those that involve the parent in delivering play therapy (Bratton, Ray, Rhine, & Jones, 2005). Several interventions for young children build on the powerful combination of the play drive and the attachment drive by having parents engage in child-led play with their children. Some of my favorites include Watch, Wait, and Wonder (WWW) (Cohen et al., 1999; Muir, Lojkasek, & Cohen, 1999), Filial Play Therapy (VanFleet, 1994), Child–Parent Psychotherapy (CPP) (Lieberman & Van Horn, 2008), and Attachment and Biobehavioral Catch-Up (ABC) (Dozier & Bernard, 2019). The positive outcomes associated with all these interventions, despite differences in specific techniques and theoretical orientations, suggest a common factor may be child-led play with a parent.

Child-Directed Interaction (CDI)

The specific type of child-led play parents are taught to provide in Integration of Working Model of Attachment into Parent–Child Interaction Therapy (IoWA-PCIT) is based on the model developed by Sheila Eyberg and is referred to as Child-Directed Interaction (CDI) (Eyberg & Funderburk, 2011; Eyberg & Matarazzo, 1980; Hembree-Kigin & McNeil, 1995; McNeil & Hembree-Kigin, 2010). CDI provides more rules and structure for how to interact with the child during child-led play than WWW, Filial Play Therapy, CPP, or ABC. Paradoxically, I find having more rules and structure makes it easier for parents to learn how to follow their child's lead in play—especially parents who did not have playful experiences during their own childhood. It is as though the structure provides the parent with the scaffolding they need in order to find their own inborn ability to play. Because there are numerous rules to CDI (reviewed in detail below), it is important for therapists to not get too caught up in the specific rules. The structure helps with teaching parents to follow their child's lead but keep your eye on the common factor—supporting the parent in following their child's lead in play.

CDI Engage and Teach Session

Prior to beginning CDI coaching sessions with the parent and child, I meet with the parents for an engage and teach session. At the engage and teach session, I go over the goals of Child-Directed Interaction (CDI) and how it will help address the child's emotional and behavioral problems. The acronym used for parents and therapists to remember the specific skills used during CDI is PRIDE. **P**raise, **R**eflect, **I**mitate, **D**escribe, and **E**njoy. CDI handouts for parents that list these skills and the reason for each skill are available at https://pcit.lab.uiowa.edu/resources/cdi-handouts.

At the engage and teach session, I let parents know that the goal of these skills is for them to enjoy spending time with their child and to learn to use specific strategies to address their child's emotional and behavioral problems. I note that many families who seek treatment no longer enjoy spending time with their child due to the constant need to manage their child's behavior and the stress this puts on the relationship. Initially, doing CDI with their child may feel like hard work as they learn new ways of interacting. However, over time, as they and their child begin doing CDI on a regular basis, they will enjoy this time with their child.

It is important to keep in mind that most parents will be surprised by the idea that playing with their child is the answer to the problems their child is experiencing. "Play with your child" is rarely on the long list of advice families have typically received prior to coming for IoWA-PCIT.

The overall goal of CDI is to follow the child's lead. As with traditional Parent–Child Interaction Therapy (PCIT), parents are learning to use their attention to modify their child's behavior. However, I never refer to the child's behavior problems as "negative attention-seeking behavior." From the perspective of attachment theory, parental attention is a need—as necessary as food or water—for a healthy childhood. My concern is that referring to the child's behavior as negative attention seeking is disparaging the child's need for attention. In addition, if I put on my behaviorist hat, I would say that we typically don't know what reinforcers the child is seeking—that is, we don't know whether the child is engaging in certain negative behaviors in order to gain attention. What we do know from attachment theory is that the need for attention from our attachment figures is a universal need. So, I focus on the power of the parents' attention to shape their child's behavior when I describe CDI to the parent.

What Parents Need from Therapists During the CDI Engage and Teach Session

The CDI engage and teach session is best conducted without the child present. Just as children learn best in a relationship where they feel valued and understood, parents learn best in a relationship where they feel valued and understood. Not having the child present allows me to focus on my relationship with the parent—establishing rapport as we discuss concerns frankly without the distraction of an active young child. The goal for this session is to communicate to the parents that I care about them as people, not just as parents.

The engage and teach session is also when I share findings of the pretreatment assessment with the parents and discuss expectations regarding how our work together will help their family. At the end of this session, I want the parent to become familiar with the skills needed to follow their child's lead in play. However, I'm not concerned about them getting all of the details of the specific skills. I know I will have lots of opportunities to scaffold the parent in these skills during the CDI coaching sessions. My primary goal is for them to leave the engage and teach session feeling hopeful about our work together and feeling that I will have their back in the process.

Just as CDI provides a structure that allows the child to lead the play, I try to provide a structure to the CDI engage and teach session that allows the parent to lead the discussion. So, although I come prepared with handouts and information from the pretreatment assessment, my goal is for this session to be a dialogue with the parent. I want this to be a discussion about the CDI skills and for the parents to feel free to raise questions and concerns about the treatment process and the specific skills. One of the ways in which I let the parent know that I am concerned about their experience is to ask them what the pretreatment observation was like for them. Parents often admit to feeling somewhat uncomfortable about being watched while they interact with their child and often note that their child was better behaved than usual. This provides me with an opportunity to validate their experience.

Parent Verbalizations Used During CDI

There are three different types of parent verbalizations the parent uses in CDI to reinforce behaviors they want to increase: Behavior description, reflection, and labeled praise. Each of these verbalizations is a different way of attending to the child's behavior. Together, they contribute to the child feeling seen (behavior description), heard (reflection), and appreciated (labeled praise) by their parent.

Behavior Description

Behavior description involves describing the child's appropriate behavior. This is the verbalization that feels the most awkward to parents and new therapists as it is not a typical way of talking to young children. A behavior description describes what the child is doing. For example, "You are putting a red block on top of the blue block" or "You are coloring on the paper." Behavior description is a way of letting the child know they are seen by the parent and plays an important role in scaffolding exploration.

Reflection

Reflection involves saying back what the child said. For example, if the child says "Doggy!" the parent gives a reflection by saying "That is a doggy!" Reflection is a way of letting the child know they are heard by the parent. Reflections also play an important role in language development. Parents of young children are often amazed at how much their child has to say once they start using reflections.

Labeled Praise

Labeled praise refers to giving the child specific praise. In other words, praise that lets the child know exactly what the parent likes about what they are doing. The best types of specific praise focus on process rather than outcome (e.g., "I like the way you are coloring so carefully" rather than "You colored a great picture"). And, the very best labeled praises are "positive opposites," that is, the opposite of the child's behavior problems. For example, if one of the parent's concerns is the child playing roughly with toys, a positive opposite praise would be "Thank you for playing gently with the toys." Labeled praise lets the child know what specific behaviors the parent appreciates. It also lets the child know the parent appreciates their efforts to engage in appropriate behavior. I also think of labeled praise as a way of expressing gratitude—letting the child know that you don't take for granted the effort it takes for a young child to sit still, play gently, use a quiet voice, and all the other behaviors we expect from young children.

Concerns About Praise

Praise is the CDI skill that evokes the most resistance from therapists and parents. Many therapists have been trained in nondirective and psychoanalytic play therapy approaches where therapists are specifically trained not to express praise, approval, or encouragement so that the child has the freedom to discover and express themselves freely. For example, in Virginia Axline's classic text on play therapy, she cautions therapists against praising children during play therapy (Axline, 1947). She describes an example of a child who was praised for being careful in the playroom. This child continued to be careful and to point out to the therapist when he was being careful. From Axline's perspective, this indicated the therapist was guiding the child's behavior during the session rather than letting the play be truly child-led.

There is no getting around the evaluative component of praise—we are encouraging the parent to explicitly tell the child what they like about the specific behaviors the child is exhibiting during Child-Directed Interaction (CDI). While I agree that nonevaluative child-led play is valuable, the truth is we do have a specific agenda when parents seek our help—enhancing the child's social-emotional functioning and improving the parent–child relationship. Telling the child explicitly what we want to see more of and acknowledging their growth and improvement is consistent with these goals. In addition, I believe praise is a powerful antidote to the history of criticism young children with disruptive behavior have often received from their parents and other adults.

Another concern expressed by therapists and parents is that children who are rewarded for behaviors will no longer be intrinsically motivated to engage in the behaviors. This concern is exemplified by research on the overjustification effect (Lepper, Greene, & Nisbett, 1973). The classic study of the overjustification effect examines the impact of giving a reward to preschool-aged children with an intrinsic interest in drawing (Lepper et al., 1973). The researchers found that the group of children who were rewarded for drawing subsequently spent less time drawing. The researchers hypothesized that by introducing a reward for drawing the child thought "I am doing this drawing *in order to* ….." (Lepper et al., 1973). In other words, they went from thinking of drawing as an activity they did because they enjoyed it to thinking of drawing as an activity they did in order to receive a reward.

As therapists who work with young children, we are especially interested in the potential risk of undermining prosocial behavior, such as the inborn tendency for altruism described in Chap. 1, by praising it. In a study of the impact of rewards on the helping behavior of young children, Werneken & Tomasello (2008) examined the impact of two types of rewards on altruism of 20-month-olds. In one condition, the adult gave the child a concrete reward for being helpful—a cube they could insert in a "jingle machine," resulting in a lovely jingling noise. In another condition, the adult praised the child for being helpful. In the control or neutral condition, the child received no reward for their altruistic behavior (helping an adult who was struggling to complete a task). Consistent with the overjustification hypothesis, children who received a concrete reward were less helpful in subsequent situations than children who received no reward.

However, praising the child for helping did not undermine the child's intrinsic motivation to behavior altruistically. Werneken & Tomasello (2008) suggest this is because praise reinforces the child's intrinsic motivation to be helpful rather than undermining it. In other words, when a child does something helpful and a parent says, "You are such a good helper for giving your baby brother the toy he dropped," the child thinks "I am a good helper" rather than thinking "I am just helping in order to get to play with the jingle machine." After reading Werneken & Tomasello's (2008) research, I was sold on the importance of using social reinforcers rather than concrete reinforcers.

Parent Nonverbal Behaviors Used During CDI

Imitation

The nonverbal behavior parents are encouraged to use during CDI is imitating the child's behavior. Imitation refers to doing what the child is doing. Mirroring or imitating their child's behavior is a powerful way for parents to connect with their child, especially for younger children.

Enjoy

The specific skills described so far provide the opportunity for what is probably the most important component of CDI—the parent enjoying spending time with their child. A caregiver's delight in their child is associated with secure attachment (Bernard & Dozier, 2011; Britner, Marvin, & Pianta, 2005). This delight is communicated through the joy parents display during interactions with their child. You can see it in the way a parent's face lights up when they look at their child, when they smile at their child, or when they snuggle back when the child sits on their lap.

It may seem obvious that enjoyment is associated with secure attachment—we all want those we love to enjoy spending time with us. But it's important to keep in mind that enjoying spending time with your child is also a high standard. Research on how much parents enjoy specific daily activities indicates parents find taking care of their children less enjoyable than socializing, watching TV, exercising, or cooking (Kahneman, Krueger, Schkade, Schwarz, & Stone, 2004).

If you have a young child with behavior problems, it isn't especially enjoyable to spend time with your child. In fact, it can be exhausting and depleting. Spending time with a child in a low-stress situation such as CDI provides the parent with a lot more opportunities to enjoy spending time with their child than they have in the course of a busy day.

Parent Verbalizations Avoided During CDI

Parents are told to avoid certain verbalizations during CDI. They are told not to criticize their child, not to give their child commands, and not to ask questions. Usually, at this point, I need to remind parents that these are rules for engaging in special play with their child, not general rules for parenting. It is difficult for most parents to imagine parenting without ever correcting their child, telling their child what to do, or asking their child questions.

Criticism

The reason for avoiding criticism during CDI seems obvious to most therapists. Being told what not to do while you're playing just isn't very fun. In the imaginative mind of a child, all kinds of things can happen during play—you can eat ice cream for breakfast and babies can fly. Yet, many parents feel the need to use play as a teaching opportunity and point out to their children that these things can't really happen.

The other reason parents criticize their child during child-led play is to manage their child's behavior. Many parents talk about their fear of raising a child who has never heard the word no—in other words, a child who does not know how to accept limits. However, many young children with disruptive behavior hear no or stop from their parents so frequently they begin to tune it out.

Commands

Avoiding commands during CDI also makes sense when we think about facilitating child-led play. Being told how to play makes the play less enjoyable. The other problem with the parent giving commands is that the child is unlikely to follow the command. By limiting the number of commands, we are also limiting the child's opportunities to fail to comply with the parent's commands.

Questions

Avoiding questions during CDI is the most difficult part of learning to provide this type of child-led play. Because it is so difficult to not ask questions, this aspect of CDI also evokes considerable resistance from therapists and parents. After all, asking questions is how most of us interact with young children—it is how we convey interest and how we find out what they're thinking and feeling.

I see parents ask a number of different types of questions during the initial evaluation and CDI sessions. It can be useful to think about these types of questions and why the parent asks them in order to have ideas about how to address them with the parent. One type of question is the "pop quiz" question. Some examples of these questions are as follows: "What color is this?" "What animal is this?" "What letter is this?" Parents often use this as a method of teaching their child—reinforcing the correct answer or correcting the child if they get the answer wrong. Although teaching the child is not the primary goal of CDI, there are ways to respect the parent's desire to teach their child and to give them an alternative approach to teaching. The parent can simply incorporate teaching into their behavior descriptions. For example, the parent can say, "You are stacking the blue block on the red block." Or, "You put the zebra and lion inside the fence." The parent can also incorporate teaching into reflections. For example, when the child labels a toy animal as a zebra, the parent can say, "You're right! That is a zebra."

Parents also frequently ask questions to express interest in their child and their child's activities. Some examples of these questions are "What did you do at school today?" "What are you building?" "What are you doing now?" "What toy do you want to play with?" It is a big shift for most parents to convey interest through behavior descriptions and reflections rather than questions. However, once they make this shift, they realize behavior descriptions and reflections are often more effective ways of conveying interest than questions.

Managing Behavior Problems During CDI

When told they are not supposed to tell their child what not to do (criticize), what to do (command), or to find out why their child is doing what they're doing (question), most parents are stumped at the idea of how they should manage their child's behavior problems during CDI. I then introduce the two behavior management strategies that will be used to manage behavior during CDI: differential attention and stopping CDI.

Differential Attention

Differential attention refers to a set of strategies that involve paying more attention to behaviors the parent wants to increase and less attention to behaviors the parent wants to decrease. Differential attention starts by praising, reflecting, describing, and imitating the positive opposites of behaviors the parent wants to decrease. The big cognitive shift the parent needs to make is *not* commenting on the behaviors they want to decrease. The parent can also make use of an active ignore where they describe their own play until the child's behavior is more appropriate.

Stopping CDI

Finally, if the child engages in dangerous or destructive behavior, the parent ends CDI. Ending CDI during a therapy appointment comes with special challenges. Ending the session because a child has engaged in the type of behavior that brought them into therapy and sending them home with a distressed parent would obviously not inspire the parent's confidence in the therapist. However, it is important that we enforce the limit during the session that we are expecting parents to enforce at home.

Therefore, I have settled on a solution that looks a bit like timing out the parent. I coach the parent to label the behavior as dangerous or destructive and inform the child that special play is over because the child engaged in the specific behavior. I then enter the room and have the parent briefly step out. Since the parent still has the communication device and I still have the microphone, the parent can hear the types of things I am saying to the child and has an idea of when I will be ready for them to reenter the room. I can also tell the parent when I am ready for them to come back into the room. When the parent comes back in the room, I typically stay in there and do CDI with them, focusing on the child's appropriate behavior.

CDI Homework

Parents are told to practice CDI at home with their child for 5 minutes each day. The positive benefits of CDI are more likely to generalize to the home if they are being practiced there. Some parents begin practicing the CDI skills with their child after they are presented in the engage and teach session. However, I typically don't start asking parents to practice CDI at home until after the first CDI coach session. Having the opportunity to coach CDI increases my confidence that CDI will be a positive experience for both parent and child once they try it at home.

Children love to play, especially with an attentive play partner. The majority of children I work with find CDI highly enjoyable and will begin asking their parent for "special play" after the parent starts practicing at home. Many parents find CDI enjoyable as well. However, finding time to do CDI competes with the numerous demands faced by parents of young children. Thus, getting parents to practice the CDI skills at home can be a struggle.

Although I strongly recommend parents practice CDI at home, I do not require parents complete CDI homework to participate in IoWA-PCIT. This is a somewhat controversial stance among more behavioral therapists who argue that the skills won't generalize if parents aren't practicing. I have given this a lot of thought, and I think it comes back to different conceptualizations of what leads to improvement in parent–child interactions. Or, as is sometimes stated in discussions of the mediating variables of interventions, what is the secret sauce that leads to improvement?

I am firmly convinced that child-led play is one of the secret sauces associated with improved functioning for young children. My years of doing individual play therapy convinced me child-led play leads to improved functioning even when the person providing the child-led play is not the parent. The power of relationships is such that a positive child-led relationship with any adult can be healing. However, my years of doing attachment-informed parent coaching convinced me that child-led play with a parent is even more powerful than child-led play with a therapist due to the importance of the parent to the child. Thus, if I have to choose between providing individual play therapy and coaching a parent in providing play therapy, I am going to coach the parent to provide play therapy—even if the parent is not practicing at home.

Managing Child's Behavior Outside of CDI

After I have gone over the details of CDI with the parent, I tell parents to continue to use their current strategies for managing their child's behavior outside of CDI. I tell parents that my role is to introduce new ways of increasing positive behavior and preventing behavior problems—not taking away strategies they are already using to manage their child's behavior problems. Many parents' experience of seeking help for concerns about their child's problems is similar to the experience of young children with behavior problems—they are told what not to do instead of what to do (e.g., don't spank, don't use time-out, he shouldn't still be using a pacifier at his age). Telling parents what not to do has the same effect on parents as it does on young children—it makes them feel negative about themselves and makes them want to defend their actions.

Parents will often ask me about how they should have responded to some crisis—for example, their child throwing themselves down in the middle of an aisle in the grocery store and throwing a tantrum. I tell parents that during a crisis they should manage the situation the best they can. I empathize with how difficult the crisis must have been for them. Parents often share thoughts about how they feel about other parents in these situations that indicate the shame they have about not being able to handle their child's behavior. The truth is I don't have great strategies for responding to crises—the nature of a crisis is that it is unpredictable. What I do have are ways of helping the parent and child learn to do better together and function better as a team, which means they will do better at weathering crises in the future.

CDI Coaching

Everything I've discussed so far is a prelude to what I consider the main event—coaching the parent in CDI. I continue to be a big believer in the power of play to help children heal—just as I was when I decided to learn individual psychoanalytic play therapy. But, over the course of my career, the research and my clinical experience have led me to view child-led play with a parent as even more powerful than child-led play with a therapist. It feels a bit like burying the lead to be discussing the most powerful part of the intervention toward the end of the chapter. I hope you have made it this far in the chapter just like I hope parents make it through the initial sessions so I have the opportunity to coach them in child-led play. As far as I'm concerned, this is where the magic happens. By focusing on the end goal and attending to parents' attachment needs during the initial sessions, I have the opportunity to coach parents of young children referred to me for behavior problems in CDI the majority of the time (95%).

What Parents Need from Therapists During CDI Coaching

During CDI coaching, parents need to be seen, heard, and appreciated. The fewer experiences the parent has with being seen, heard, and appreciated, the more they will need to experience this with us before they can provide this for their child. During CDI coaching, we do this by making observations about their importance to their child. For example, noting how their child looks at them for approval. We also let them know that we appreciate them by praising their efforts during CDI. The vast majority of my statements during CDI coaching (80–95%) are positive, responsive statements. In other words, most of my statements point out something positive the parent said or did during their interactions with their child.

Tracking Progress in CDI

By spending a few minutes on assessment at the beginning of each CDI session, we are able to tailor our coaching to current strengths and concerns. We are also able to track progress over time by using standardized assessments and observations. There are two sources of information we use for these assessments: (1) parent ratings of disruptive behavior and (2) 5 minutes of observation at the beginning of the CDI session.

Parent Ratings of Disruptive Behavior

At the beginning of the Child-Directed Interaction (CDI) sessions, I have the parent complete the Eyberg Child Behavior Inventory (ECBI) (Eyberg & Pincus, 1999). Many of the therapists I train have begun using an alternative to the ECBI at the beginning of CDI sessions called the Weekly Assessment of Child Behavior–Positive (WACB-P) (Forte, Boys, & Timmer, 2012). The advantage of the WACB-P is that it is free and has fewer questions than the ECBI. The WACB-P is available at https://pcit.ucdavis.edu/forms/cdi-forms/.

Observations of Parent–Child Interactions

After the parent has completed the ECBI or WACB-P, there is an observation of the parent and child engaging in CDI. I let the parent know through the communication device that I will be observing for a few minutes and then will give them some feedback and coach. I aim to observe for 5 minutes, but I am alert to the possibility that I may not make it through 5 minutes of observation if the interactions become extremely negative or the child engages in dangerous or destructive behavior. During the 5 minutes of observation, I am coding parent verbalizations using the Dyadic Parent–Child Interaction Coding System (DPICS) (Eyberg, Nelson, Ginn, Bhuiyan, & Boggs, 2013), just as I did at the pretreatment evaluation. I am also observing the child's response to the parent's use of the PRIDE skills. Finally, I am observing how the parent supports the child's needs for attachment and exploration. While doing this, I am staying alert to the possibility that I may need to cut the observation short and begin coaching. Examples of situations that lead me to jump in and start coaching before finishing the 5 minutes of observation are as follows: (1) the child engaging in dangerous or destructive behavior, (2) the parent being extremely critical and giving a lot of commands, and (3) the parent becoming extremely upset with the child. Yes—there is a lot to pay attention to during this 5-minute observation.

If I have been able to code for 5 minutes, I tell the parent to let the child know that the parent will be listening to me for a minute while the child continues to play. There are a couple of reasons why I have parents give this notification to the child. First, it seems only fair to me that the child knows why their parent has gone from giving them undivided attention to withdrawing their attention. By letting their child know they are listening to me they communicate clearly the reason for withdrawing their attention. Second, it is the beginning of the parent being able to calmly state a transition—the beginning of teaching the child to accept a limit. Here is a specific example of what I might say at the end of coding.

Therapist to parent: "Tell Sally-Jane that you're going to listen to me for a minute while she plays."
Parent to child: "I'm going to listen to the doctor for a minute while you play."
Child to parent: "OK."

Therapist to parent: "Great job of letting Sally-Jane know what's going to happen next. And she accepted it! You did an amazing job of following her lead today. I can see how much she loves this time with you. I loved how gentle and careful she was with the baby dolls. Sharing your attention with me now will be tough for her so I'll try to be fast. You had lots of PRIDE skills today—4 labeled praises, 7 reflections, and 2 behavior descriptions. You still are asking a few questions but you only gave one command and there was no negative talk. Sally-Jane has done a great job of playing quietly while you listened to me. Go ahead and praise her for playing quietly and then go back to those excellent CDI skills."
Parent to child: "Thanks for playing quietly so I could listen to the doctor."
Child to parent: "What did she say?"
Therapist to parent: "You can tell Sally-Jane that I was telling you how impressed I was with how gently she was playing with the toys today."
Parent to child: "Doctor Beth was telling me she noticed how gentle you were with her babies."

Coaching CDI in the Family's Home

The majority of my experience conducting CDI is in the clinic where I have a playroom, specific toys, and specialized equipment for coaching parents through a communication device. Over the course of the COVID-19 pandemic, I have gained experience in coaching CDI in the family's home over telehealth. There are challenges to coaching CDI in the family's home, but I began to see the benefits of this approach as well. Let me start with the benefits. This experience reminded me of my research experiences assessing newborns in their home. There is something about being invited into someone's home that immediately creates a bond. I felt like I got to know parents and children a bit faster when they invited me into their home via telehealth. I also had an opportunity to see where they would be practicing CDI at home and to see the types of toys they would be using in CDI. I found this useful in helping parents generalize the skills and in evaluating challenges to practicing the CDI skills at home.

One of the things I learned early on was how different the child's exploration looks when coaching CDI in the family's home. When coaching parents in the clinic, a new setting with novel toys, the child's exploration typically focuses on exploring the playroom. When I coach parents in their home via telehealth, I find children have a larger range of exploration—much of it happening "off camera" for me. Children will run to another room to get a toy, get up and follow a cat that walked through the session, or leave to find out what another family member is doing. I learned to become more comfortable with this wider range of exploration and to recognize it as part of the healthy attachment–exploration balance we see in secure attachment. When the child's exploration takes them off camera, I check in with the parent to make sure they are okay with the child's exploration and use the time to talk with the parent about any questions or concerns. Then, I have the parent pick up a toy and describe what they are doing (as we do in an active ignore) until the child returns to play with them.

Perhaps because everyone was so socially isolated at the beginning of the COVID-19 pandemic, I also found children were sometimes more interested in interacting with me than their parent during telehealth sessions. I addressed this by trying to create check-in and check-out routines similar to the routines that are part of CDI sessions in the clinic. During a brief check-in at the beginning of the session, the child showed me their toys while I did CDI with them. For example, "You're showing me a blue block. Thank you for showing me the toys you and your mom are going to play with today." During a brief check-out at the end of the session, I gave the child labeled praise for their behavior during the session before ending. Learning to do CDI coaching via telehealth reminded me to keep my eye on the core component of the intervention, the power of attachment and play, during a time when we needed both.

Determining How Long to Continue the CDI Phase

The parent and child continue in the CDI phase until several goals are met: (1) The parent–child relationship has improved to the point where the parent and child clearly enjoy spending time together during CDI. (2) The parent is engaging in the PRIDE skills at a very high rate during CDI. I use the specific mastery criteria used in traditional PCIT to evaluate this (i.e., 10 labeled praise, 10 reflections, and 10 behavior descriptions during the 5 minutes of coding at the beginning of the CDI session). (3) The parent is rarely criticizing, giving commands, or asking questions during CDI. Again, I use the specific mastery criteria used in traditional PCIT to evaluate this [i.e., the parent gives three or fewer negative leading statements (negative talk, questions, or commands) during the 5 minutes of CDI coding]. (4) The parent is managing the child's misbehavior through the use of differential attention. Finally, (5) the parent is responsive to my coaching.

The Bottom Line

Teaching parents to follow their child's lead in play builds on children's inborn desire to be in relationship and their inborn desire to play. The combination of these powerful factors can be a significant impetus for improving parent–child interactions and social-emotional functioning. Because children are at their best when playing with their parents, we have opportunities to build on the child's capacity for prosocial skills, regulation, and positive interactions with their parent. We also have multiple opportunities to reinforce what is going well in the relationship through our in-the-moment coaching, providing the parent with the type of positive experience they are providing for their child.

References

Axline, V. (1947). *Play therapy: The inner dynamics of childhood*. Houghton Mifflin Company.

Bernard, K., & Dozier, M. (2011). This is my baby: Foster parents' feelings of commitment and displays of delight. *Infant Mental Health Journal, 32*(2), 251–262.

Bratton, S., Ray, E., Rhine, T., & Jones, L. (2005). The efficacy of play therapy with children: A meta-analytic review of treatment outcomes. *Professional Psychology: Research and Practice, 36*(4), 376–390.

Britner, P., Marvin, R., & Pianta, R. (2005). Development and preliminary validation of the caregiving behavior system: Association with child attachment classification in the preschool strange situation. *Attachment & Human Development, 7*, 83–102.

Cohen, N., Muir, E., Lojkasek, M., Muir, R., Parker, C., Barwick, M., & Brown, M. (1999). Watch, wait and wonder: Testing the effectiveness of a new approach to mother-infant psychotherapy. *Infant Mental Health Journal, 20*, 429–451.

Dozier, M., & Bernard, K. (2019). *Coaching parents of vulnerable infants: The attachment and biobehavioral catch-up approach*. The Guilford Press.

Eyberg, S., & Funderburk, B. (2011). *Parent-child interaction therapy protocol*. PCIT International, Inc.

Eyberg, S., & Matarazzo, R. (1980). Training parents as therapists: A comparison between individual parent-child interaction training and parent group didactic training. *Journal of Clinical Psychology, 36*, 492–499.

Eyberg, S., & Pincus, D. (1999). *Eyberg child behavior inventory and sutter-eyberg student behavior inventory - revised*. Psychological Assessment Resources.

Eyberg, S., Nelson, M., Ginn, N., Bhuiyan, N., & Boggs, S. (2013). *Dyadic Parent-Child Interaction Coding System (DPICS): Comprehensive manual for research and training*. PCIT International, Inc..

Forte, L., Boys, D., & Timmer, S. (2012). *The use of child behavior assessments for weekly check-ins in PCIT: WACB-N and WACB-P*. Paper presented at the 12th Annual PCIT Conference for Traumatized Children.

Gray, P. (2009). Play as a foundation for hunter-gatherer social existence. *American Journal of Play, 1*, 476–522.

Gray, P. (2011). The decline of play and the rise of psychopathology in children and adolescents. *American Journal of Play, 3*, 443–463.

Gray, P. (2013). The value of a play-filled childhood in development of the hunter-gatherer individual. In N. Darcia, J. Panksepp, A. Schore, & T. Gleason (Eds.), *Evolution, early experience and human development: From research to practice and policy* (pp. 352–370). Oxford University Press.

Hembree-Kigin, T., & McNeil, C. (1995). *Parent-child interaction therapy*. Plenum Press.

Kahneman, D., Krueger, A., Schkade, D., Schwarz, N., & Stone, A. (2004). A Survey method for characterizing daily life experience: The day reconstruction method. *Science, 306*(5702), 1776–1780.

Lepper, M., Greene, D., & Nisbett, R. (1973). Undermining children's intrinsic interest with extrinsic reward: A test of the "Overjustification" hypothesis. *Journal of Personality and Social Psychology, 28*(1), 129–137.

Lieberman, A., & Van Horn, P. (2008). *Psychotherapy with infants and young children: Repairing the effects of stress and trauma on early attachment*. The Guilford Press.

McNeil, C., & Hembree-Kigin, T. (2010). *Parent-child interaction therapy* (2nd ed.). Springer.

Muir, E., Lojkasek, M., & Cohen, N. (1999). *Watch, wait, & wonder: A manual describing a dyadic infant-led approach to problems in infancy and early childhood*. Hincks-Dellcrest Institute.

VanFleet, R. (1994). *Filial therapy: Strengthening parent-child relationships through play*. Professional Resource Press.

Werneken, F., & Tomasello, M. (2008). Extrinsic rewards undermine altruistic tendencies in 20-month-olds. *Developmental Psychology, 44*(6), 1758–1788.

Chapter 5
How to Coach Parents to Set Limits and Improve Child Compliance

This chapter addresses how to coach parents through one of the most challenging aspects of parenting a young child—setting limits. I discuss the role of limit-setting in healthy attachment relationships. I describe how to use Parent-Directed Interaction (PDI) to teach parents to set limits and improve child compliance. I also describe how to present Parent-Directed Interaction (PDI) to parents and how to talk with parents about their feelings and concerns regarding discipline. I describe how to coach parents in setting limits with their child using PDI, how to explain PDI to the child, and how to gradually introduce this disciplinary procedure in the home.

Parent-Directed Interaction (PDI)

Teaching parents to set limits is the focus of the second phase of Integration of Working Models of Attachment into Parent–Child Interaction Therapy (IoWA-PCIT). Parents are first taught how to increase their child's compliance with commands during a relatively low-stress situation. Parents are then taught how to improve compliance and set limits on their child's behavior in more challenging situations. The parent is coached in specific skills for responding to compliance and noncompliance—in ways that increase compliance and reduce the stress and anxiety associated with responding to their child's misbehavior and noncompliance.

The specific skills taught in the PDI phase of IoWA-PCIT are based on the skills taught in other versions of PCIT (Eyberg & Funderburk, 2011; Eyberg & Matarazzo, 1980; Hembree-Kigin & McNeil, 1995; McNeil & Hembree-Kigin, 2010; Urquiza, Zebell, Timmer, & McGrath, 2012). IoWA-PCIT includes some modifications to make the PDI protocol and PDI coaching more consistent with attachment theory. PDI handouts for parents are available at https://pcit.lab.uiowa.edu/resources/pdi-handouts.

The development of the PDI phase of IoWA-PCIT was also informed by the attachment-informed research on sensitive discipline for young children (Van Zeijl, Mesman, Van Ijzendoorn, Bakermans-Kranenburg, Juffer, Stolk et al., 2006). "Video-feedback Intervention to promote Positive Parenting and Sensitive Discipline" (VIPP-SD) (Van Zeijl et al., 2006) provided me with an example of how parents could use a time-out procedure in a manner that was sensitive to the attachment needs of young children. VIPP-SD is an adaptation of "Video-feedback Intervention to promote Positive Parenting and Sensitive Discipline" (VIPP), which was developed to address the needs of young children with disruptive behavior. Like other versions of VIPP, VIPP-SD emphasizes using video feedback to reinforce parents' responsiveness to the attachment cues of their child. VIPP-SD also emphasizes the importance of co-regulation in soothing young children's distress. It also describes how parents can set limits and use time-out in a way that is sensitive to the child's wishes and needs while providing clear boundaries and consequences. This research reassured me that attachment theory and the use of time-out were not incompatible. This research also alerted me to one of our most important roles when coaching parents through setting limits—how to be sensitive to the child's feelings while providing clear consequences.

Importance of Limit-Setting in Healthy Attachment

There are a number of ways in which parents need to be "bigger, stronger, wiser, and kind" (Powell, Cooper, Hoffman, & Marvin, 2014) in order to be effective parents. Young children need their parents to guide their behavior. Teaching a child to follow directions is an important step in being able to guide a child's behavior. Sometimes, in current conceptualizations of attachment theory, parents and therapists have shifted the balance to a primary focus on responding to the child's attachment needs, omitting or downplaying limit-setting. It seems like the need for parents to set limits and help their child learn to accept limits is sometimes overlooked. So, prior to diving into the details of PDI, I discuss with parents the importance of limit-setting in healthy attachment development and healthy social-emotional development, especially as infants transition to toddlers and preschoolers.

In her first book on attachment, *Infancy in Uganda*, Mary Ainsworth (1967) tackles the question of when parents should begin setting limits. "There is a point, however, toward the end of the first year of life or early in the second year, when a baby's confidence in being able to control his world through his own actions is well enough established that parents can begin to show him the limits of his power." According to Ainsworth (1967), "It may be difficult to judge when the time has come to begin to demonstrate to an infant the limits of his power, but sooner or later—yet not too soon—he must learn that he is not king and cannot control his parents at his whim. He must find out, perhaps largely through trial and error, just what he can control and what he cannot control, and what he can influence by the right techniques but cannot be sure of controlling."

There are clear parallels between Ainsworth's (1967) description of how children learn to accept limits and the two phases of IoWA-PCIT. In the first phase, Child-Directed Interaction (CDI) (described in Chap. 4), there is a clear emphasis on responding to the child's needs by following their lead—similar to the sensitive responsive parenting in the first year of life associated with secure attachment. In the second phase (PDI), the emphasis turns to helping the child accept limits.

Research on Limit-Setting and Secure Attachment

Ainsworth's observations about the importance of limit-setting in healthy attachment have been supported by research on attachment theory. According to attachment researchers Howard and Miriam Steele, "The child whose aggression is not safely limited will be vulnerable to unlimited aggressive impulses" (Steele & Steele, 2005). This quote is from a chapter describing a longitudinal study that found strong support for the association of secure attachment and limit-setting (Steele & Steele, 2005). Steele and Steele (2005) interviewed mothers during pregnancy using the Adult Attachment Interview (AAI) (George, Kaplan, & Main, 1984; Main, 2000). Then, when children of these mothers were 5 years old, Steele and Steele (2005) assessed the children's working model of attachment. They found that "the most powerful finding to emerge from statistical analyses was the significantly elevated levels of limit-setting responses (e.g., most commonly evident when children depicted a parent who exercised authority with verbal discipline) among children whose mothers had provided autonomous-secure AAIs more than 5 years previously, before the birth of the children" (Steele & Steele, 2005).

In other words, 5-year-olds raised by mothers with secure/autonomous attachment know where the boundaries are. These young children had internalized a sense of how a parent would respond to misbehavior. In the stories told by children with secure mothers, parents were firm and clearly communicated their expectations when norms were violated.

In IoWA-PCIT, our goal when teaching parents to set limits with their children in PDI is similar. First, we teach parents to clearly communicate expectations to their child. Second, we teach parents to use—and communicate—consistent, predictable responses to violations of these expectations.

It seems like discipline has a bad reputation with therapists and parents in recent years, perhaps because the term has become associated with punitive and coercive techniques that conjure up distressing memories of childhood. I sometimes talk with parents about how the root of the word discipline means to teach and that effective discipline teaches the child important life lessons. The most important lesson the child learns in the PDI phase of treatment is to follow directions.

I talk with parents about how we are going to teach their child to follow directions by breaking the task down into small, teachable moments. As noted by Ainsworth (1967), children often learn the limits of their control through trial and error. Thus, it should not be a surprise that so many children struggle to learn this lesson. In PDI, the consequences are extremely predictable, making it easier for the child to learn the task of following directions. The metaphor I often use with parents is that teaching children to follow directions and accept consequences for their actions is similar to teaching children to read. When we are teaching children to read, we break it down into smaller steps to make it easy and fun for them to read. We start with teaching them their ABCs through a song. We then progress to reading to them and sharing picture books with a few words. Once they have learned to sound out words and enjoy reading, we are able to share chapter books.

In the same way we break down learning to read for young children, we break down learning to follow directions in the PDI phase of IoWA-PCIT. My colleague Tracy Vozar has suggested we call this phase PDI + CDI in order to emphasize that CDI is still an important component of this phase of intervention. In fact, it might be even more accurate to call it PDI + lots of CDI. Just as attachment theory emphasizes the role of a healthy attachment relationship in teaching children boundaries and limits, IoWA-PCIT emphasizes the role of CDI as a prerequisite to teaching children to listen and follow directions.

Eight Rules of Effective Commands in PDI

The first part of the PDI phase of IoWA-PCIT involves teaching parents to give effective commands. The eight rules of effective commands are a component of other models of PCIT (Eyberg & Funderburk, 2011; Eyberg & Matarazzo, 1980; Eyberg & Pincus, 1999; Hembree-Kigin & McNeil, 1995; McNeil & Hembree-Kigin, 2010). The acronym I use for the eight rules of effective commands is PRACTICE. **P**ositively state the command, **R**eason before command and/or after compliance, **A**ge-appropriate command, **C**alm and courteous command, **T**ell, don't ask, **I**ndividual command, **C**lear command, **E**nough commands.

There are a couple of reasons why I created the acronym PRACTICE to help parents and therapists remember the rules of effective commands in PDI. First, the PRACTICE acronym reminds parents that learning to follow directions is a new skill that requires practice. Second, the PRACTICE acronym reminds parents that as they are beginning to give PDI commands at home it is helpful to tell the child "It is time to practice listening."

Positively State the Command

The first rule of effective commands is to give a command that is positively stated—in other words, commands that tell children what to do rather than what not to do. For example, if a child is standing on a chair, telling them "Please get off the chair" is a positively stated command because it tells them what to do rather than what not to do.

Reason Before Command and/or After Compliance

The second rule is to give a reason for the command before giving the command. We all do better with following commands if we understand the reason for the command. Perhaps because I have some oppositional leanings, I am amazed by the vast majority of children who follow hundreds of commands each day without knowing the reason for them. My heart is with the oppositional children who want to know the reason they are being told to do something. At the initial phase of PDI, the reason parents give their child for a command is "It's time to practice listening." As stated earlier, learning to follow directions is treated as a skill that needs to be learned by the child and like any skill it needs to be practiced. By telling the child "It's time to practice listening" before giving a command, the parent reminds the child (and the parent) of the importance of learning to practice the skill of learning to follow directions.

If parents forget to give a reason before giving a command, they should give the reason after the child has complied with the command. However, they should not give the reason when the child asks, "Why do I have to get off the chair?" or "Why do I have to practice listening?" The problem with giving the reason in response to the child asking why they have to do something is the parent is then put in a position of coming up with a good enough reason to get the child to comply. For example, a common answer to "Why do I have to get off the chair?" is "Because you might fall." The child then answers, "No, I won't." This puts the parent in the position of coming up with a better reason such as "It's hard on the chair." And, of course, the child's answer is, "No, it's not." You get the drift of how long this argument can continue as the parent tries to talk the child into following directions.

Age-Appropriate Command

The third rule is to give a command that is age appropriate. Children make such huge changes in the first few years of life that it is easy to forget how recently they have acquired language and motor skills. Following directions involves understanding the parent's command, deciding whether to comply, and coordinating the motor skills involved in complying with the command. The process of complying can break down at any step in this process. Although parents of young oppositional children typically assume the process breaks down at the decision to comply stage, I'm struck during initial evaluations at how many commands parents give where it is literally not possible for a young child to comply.

Calm and Courteous Command

The fourth rule is to give a command that is calm and courteous. I encourage parents to start the command with "Please" as a way of modeling politeness. I tell parents that I know children train parents to yell. Basically, young children with attention problems tend not to pay attention until the parent raises their voice. This leads to a cycle where the parent finds they are yelling more and becoming more upset over time in their attempts to get their child to listen. The goal of PDI is to retrain their child to follow directions when the parent is calm, polite, and kind.

Tell, Don't Ask

The fifth rule is to tell the child what to do rather than asking them to do something. This is referred to as a direct command in the behavioral parenting literature. This rule involves a bit of unpacking and discussion. Most of us prefer asking a child to do something rather than telling them to do it—it seems more polite to ask if they would like to pick up their toys instead of telling them to pick up their toys. I find it can help to have an analogy when thinking through the reason for giving children direct commands when we are teaching them to comply with directions. Let's say your boss asks you if you would like to spend the long weekend you had planned to spend at the beach working on a project. You politely say "No Thank You" to his question as you know the project isn't due for a couple of weeks and had your heart set on beach time. When performance review time comes around, your boss gives you a negative review for failing to work over the long weekend. Does this seem fair? Of course not! Young children with oppositional tendencies can feel the same way about requests. When asked if they want to pick up the toys, go to bed, or any number of requests that are less fun than a beach vacation, they are likely to decline the offer. Then, when they receive a negative consequence, they are stunned. How unfair! They gave an honest answer and were punished.

Because we teach parents to use direct commands as part of the process of teaching children to comply with commands, there is a common misunderstanding that direct commands are better than indirect commands for young children. This is not always the case. When children follow indirect commands (suggestions or requests), they are internalizing the parent's values, a type of compliance referred to as "committed compliance" (Kochanska, 2002).

I think of direct commands as part of the clear communication aspect of secure attachment. A direct command signals to the child when they need to comply and there is no room for negotiation (e.g., getting off that fragile dining room chair they are standing on at your in-law's home). There are still plenty of times when parents may choose to give indirect commands.

Individual Command

The sixth rule is to give a single command rather than multiple commands. At pretreatment, a parent telling their child to pick up toys can sound something like this: "Pick up all the toys and put them away. Would you please pick up the toys? No—not like that. Be careful with the toys. Let's pick up the blocks now. Why don't you want to pick up the toys?" Part of what we do in PDI is to slow the process down so the child has the chance to comply with each individual command. For example, an early clean-up command might be, "It's almost time to go. Please put this block in the box." If you've ever had to clean up your house after a great party or clean up your office after writing a big grant, you know how overwhelming the task of clean-up can be. By giving the child a single command, we break the process down into a manageable task for the child. This type of scaffolding helps the child feel successful at listening and cleaning up. The other advantage of single commands is there are multiple opportunities to praise the child for compliance.

Clear Command

The seventh rule is to give a clear command. Again, since one of the hallmarks of secure attachment is clear communication, this is consistent with attachment theory. Also, we want to ensure the parent gives a command where we can clearly judge whether the child has complied. To make it even more explicit, we indicate the child must be able to comply with the command in the immediate future (i.e., within 5 seconds) in order for the command to count as a clear command.

Enough Commands

The eighth rule is to give enough commands. For many parents, this means learning to limit the number of commands they give their child. Sometimes, at this point in treatment, I will share with parents the number of commands they gave their child at the pretreatment evaluation. They are often stunned to hear they gave their child more than 50 commands in 10 minutes at the initial evaluation. They realize it is unrealistic to expect anyone, but especially a young child, to follow that many commands.

For other parents, giving enough commands means they need to learn how to give their child enough commands for their child to have practice in following commands and accepting limits. These are parents who have too few expectations for their child. This type of parenting has been characterized as permissive parenting (Baumrind, 1966), that is, high nurturance but few limits. The other group of parents who need to be encouraged to give enough commands are those who, because of their child's history of noncompliance, have quit giving their child commands—much as you might quit telling your child to tie their shoes if they hadn't learned how to tie them.

If you're thinking this is a lot of rules. You're right. It is. It turns out that the secret to getting children to follow rules is teaching their parents a lot of specific rules that set their child up for success in learning to follow directions. When teaching parents to set limits, I think therapists can easily fall into the trap of placing too much emphasis on the "back end" —that is, what to do when the child has failed to follow directions or has engaged in aggressive or destructive behavior. It turns out that by focusing on the "front end"—teaching parents how to clearly communicate expectations—we can significantly increase compliance. Parents will learn to give commands that follow these rules by being coached in giving effective commands.

Response to Compliance

The next rule parents learn in teaching their child to follow commands is how to respond to compliance and noncompliance. One of the hardest rules for many parents to learn is to wait quietly for compliance. After a parent has given a command, I tell them to wait quietly for up to 5 seconds to see whether their child is going to follow the command. Five seconds is not that long for children to comprehend a command, decide on whether they are going to comply, and either choose to comply with the command or not. However, from the perspective of a parent, 5 seconds can feel like a very long time. Again, although the ultimate focus of our parent coaching is teaching children to be patient, it turns out that teaching parents to be patient is part of the process that gets us to that goal.

If the child follows the command, the parent gives the child labeled praise for compliance. For example, "Thank you for following directions." Because parents have become skilled at giving specific praise by the time we get to this phase of treatment, parents are often very specific in their praise—for example, "Thank you for handing me the yellow block." It is great to give this type of specific praise but we also want parents to praise the class of behaviors we are focusing on increasing—that is, compliance. So, it is important parents also give specific praises like "I appreciate you doing what I told you to do," "Great first time listening," and "I am so proud of you for being a good listener."

Response to Noncompliance

If the child fails to follow the command within 5 seconds, the parent gives the child a warning about the consequence of failing to follow directions. The standard warning is, "If you don't _____ (the parent repeats the original command), you'll have to sit on the time-out chair" (Eyberg & Funderburk, 2011;

McNeil & Hembree-Kigin, 2010). The parent then waits another 5 seconds for the child to comply with the command. (As part of tailoring PDI, there may be times when you modify the consequence for noncompliance.)

If the child fails to follow the command following the time-out warning, the parent will escort the child to the time-out chair. Some children are willing and able to walk to the time-out chair when the parent stands up and points to the chair. However, some young children need to be carried to the time-out chair by the parent. If the child needs to be carried to the time-out chair, it is recommended the parent pick up the child from behind underneath the arms. This is the safest carry for both the parent and child.

I recommend using an adult-size chair with arms as the time-out chair. The time-out chair should be placed far enough away from walls that the child cannot hit or kick the walls while on the time-out chair. I prefer the time-out chair be faced into the room, not into a corner. This allows the child to see the parent while they are on the time-out chair.

It is important to remember that most of the children we are working with in IoWA-PCIT are at the stage of attachment development where they have a goal-corrected partnership with their parent (Ainsworth, Blehar, Waters, & Wall, 1978; Bowlby, 1969). That is, both the parent and child have their own agenda and are trying to influence their partner to go along with their agenda. When we're coaching parents through PDI, it is important to recognize this. That is, children have a right to their own agenda and are way more flexible in their attempts to influence their parent's agenda than we might expect. But parents have both a right and a responsibility to set the agenda and enforce boundaries.

One of my favorite child development studies is a study of tool use in toddlers called *Out of the Toolbox: Toddlers Differentiate Wobbly and Wooden Handrails* (Berger, Adolph, & Lobo, 2005). The purpose of the study was to examine the development of tool use by examining how 16-month-old toddlers assessed the effectiveness of different types of handrails in crossing a bridge. The handrails were either "wobbly" (made out of foam or latex) or sturdy wooden handrails. As predicted, the toddlers made more attempts to cross the bridge when provided with study wooden handrails. The unanticipated finding, and my favorite part of the study, was the number of toddlers who figured out a way to cross the bridge using the *wobbly* handrails. In the words of the researchers, "Infants' high success rate with wobbly handrails was due to the inventiveness of their problem solving (and a failure on the part of the experimenters to anticipate such ingenuity)" (Berger et al., 2005). Examples of successful strategies included hunching over the handrails and walking sideways, distributing their weight between the handrails, and pulling themselves across the bridge using the wobbly handrails as a rope.

I think of this study often when coaching PDI. Young children are way more flexible thinkers than adults. They come up with very creative responses to our very predictable and rigid system of how to respond to compliance and noncompliance. While I marvel at the cognitive flexibility of young children and rather enjoy watching the different strategies they use, I also recognize that they need the sturdiness and predictability of solid handrails on their bridge to independence.

There are a few inventive strategies that happen often enough in PDI that it is worth reviewing them so you can be prepared and know how to coach parents to respond in a predictable way in the face of their child's inventive strategies. An inventive strategy I see frequently is children who follow a slightly different command than the command that was given. For example, the parent tells the child to hand her a block and the child hands her a doll instead. Although I admire the child's ingenuity, it is important to have the parent treat this as noncompliance during PDI practice. The parent needs to stick with the PDI script and give the time-out warning for this type of partial compliance.

Some children respond to being given a time-out warning by "putting themself in time-out." That is, when the parent says, "If you don't _____, you'll have to sit on the time-out chair." The child says, "I'm not listening, and I'll just put myself in time-out." The child then walks to the time-out chair and sits on the chair. To the child, this seems like an effective strategy for undercutting the parent's and therapist's authority by indicating they don't care about the consequence. If this happens, the parent goes ahead and follows the PDI script by stating, "You didn't do what I told you to do so you have to sit on the time-out chair."

I have also seen young children use a similar strategy after complying with a command and being praised for compliance—returning to sit on the time-out chair after following a command instead of playing with the parent. Since the parent doesn't need to follow the PDI script in this case (since the child has complied), the parent can play by themselves while describing their own play, just as they do during an active ignore, until the child is ready to come play with them.

An inventive strategy that is especially challenging for parents and therapists is when the child complies on the way to the time-out chair. Once the parent has said the child has to sit on the time-out chair, it is important the parent follow through with the time-out. In effect, telling the child to sit on the time-out chair is the last and most important command at this point. Having the child comply with taking a time-out, even when it feels unfair to the child (and possibly to us), will ultimately result in fewer time-outs. Remember that our goal is for children to comply earlier in the sequence (i.e., after the command or the time-out warning). Learning that complying too late does not count as compliance is a tough lesson. But it is a lesson I typically see children learn on the first try.

Response to Getting Off Time-Out Chair and Unsafe Behavior on Time-Out Chair

We need to ensure the child stays on the time-out chair and sits safely on the time-out chair in order for time-out to be a safe and effective consequence. Thus, there needs to be a consequence for getting off the time-out chair and for unsafe behavior on the time-out chair (e.g., standing on the chair, rocking the chair, and scooting the chair). The consequence for getting off the time-out chair varies between the different PCIT protocols (Eyberg & Funderburk, 2011; Hembree-Kigin & McNeil, 1995; McNeil & Hembree-Kigin, 2010; Urquiza et al., 2012), reflecting the evolution of PDI and the particular challenges associated with finding an appropriate backup consequence. Before discussing the backup consequences I use in PDI, I want to share a bit of this evolution.

The backup consequences used in previous PDI protocols include a spank (Hembree-Kigin & McNeil, 1995), placement in an empty room (Eyberg & Funderburk, 2011; McNeil & Hembree-Kigin, 2010; Urquiza et al., 2012), and loss of a privilege (Urquiza et al., 2012). It is shocking for most therapists (myself included) to consider a time when spanking was condoned by early-childhood therapists. In fact, this aspect of PCIT was a primary factor in my objection to this model early in my career. I think it is important to be familiar with the history of any therapeutic approach and to be aware of the extent to which it is tied to the era when it was developed. Spanking was considered a common and acceptable child-rearing practice in the 1970s when PCIT and other behavioral parent training interventions were developed and, by introducing the use of a time-out procedure, PCIT likely reduced the use of spanking by parents.

By 2007, when I began disseminating PCIT in Iowa, spanking was no longer considered an appropriate backup consequence. Instead, the backup consequence used was 1 minute alone in a room. Consistent with other versions of PCIT (Eyberg & Funderburk, 2011; McNeil & Hembree-Kigin, 2010; Urquiza et al., 2012), this is the backup consequence I use most often. The majority of parents I work with in IoWA-PCIT are sending their child to their room for misbehavior at the beginning of treatment. So, I am typically introducing specific circumstances for sending their child to their room rather than recommending a new discipline procedure. Sometimes, the backup consequence I use is the loss of a privilege, a consequence used in the PCIT for Traumatized Children protocol (PCIT-TC) (Urquiza et al., 2012). When using this backup, the child loses access to some preferred object or activity (decided on ahead of time) until they complete their time-out and comply with the command.

Explaining PDI to the Child: Coaching Parent Through Explanation

At the initial PDI session, it seems only fair to let the child know that the session is going to be a bit different and that expectations have changed. Some parents will have talked with the child about PDI prior to the initial PDI session. I have the parent explain PDI again during the session even if the parent has explained it prior to the session. There are a variety of different ways the PDI process can be explained to the child. Typically, I talk the parent through explaining the process to the child. The explanation I have the parent give sounds something like this: "Today is going to be a little different. Today you're going to practice listening. It's really important that you learn to listen and follow directions. I'm going to tell you things to do. If you do what I tell you to do, we'll get to keep playing. If you don't do what I tell you to do, you'll have to sit on the time-out chair. If you have to sit on the time-out chair, you need to sit there until I say you can get off. If you get off the chair before I say you can, you will have to go to another room without toys (or I will take the toys and wait outside)."

When talking the parent through this, the goal is to tell the parent exactly what to say a line at a time. The goal is to have the parent matter-of-factly explain the process to the child. Ideally, you want the parent to get through the explanation without giving commands or arguing with the child. You also want to avoid having the child derail the explanation. In reality, it often sounds something like this.

Therapist to parent: "Tell Janey that today is going to be little different."
Parent to child: "Janey, today is going to be a little different."
Child to parent: "OK."
Therapist to parent: "Today you're going to practice listening."
Parent to child: "Today you're going to practice listening."
Therapist to parent: "It's really important that you learn to listen and follow directions."
Parent to child: "It's really important that you learn to listen and follow directions."
Child to parent: "I don't like that idea."
Child shakes head no.
Parent to child: "I'm going to tell you things to do. If you do them, we'll get to keep playing."
Child stacks blocks and ignores parent.
Parent to child: "Pay attention Janey. Listen to me."
Therapist to child: "That's okay. You don't need to make sure she is paying attention. I'm going to keep telling you how to explain it to her. Tell her "If you don't do what I tell you to do, you'll have to sit on the time-out chair."
Parent to child: "If you don't do what I tell you to do, you'll have to sit on the time-out chair."
Child to parent: Briefly pauses stacking blocks, looks at her mother, and says, "No chair."
Therapist to parent: "Tell her if you need to sit on the time-out chair, you need to sit there until I tell you to get off."
Parent to child: "If we need to go to time-out."
Therapist to parent: "Say if **you** need to sit on the time-out chair, you need to sit there until I tell you to get off."
Parent to child: "If you need to sit on the time-out chair, you need to sit there until I tell you to get off."
Child to parent: Goes over to table and begins coloring.
Therapist to parent: "Tell her if you get off the chair before I say you can, you'll have to go to another room without toys."
Parent to child: "If you get off the chair before I say you can, you'll have to go to another room without toys."

Therapist to parent: "OK. Now you can do CDI with her for a couple of minutes and I'll tell you when to give the first command. Go join her at the table and describe what she is doing."

Explaining PDI to the Child: Therapist Explanation

The therapist may prefer to explain PDI directly to the child. This allows the therapist to have more control of the process, moving through the explanation quickly and ignoring objections from the child. This also provides a review of the PDI procedure for the parent. The therapist may choose to use props such as a stuffed animal to demonstrate PDI to the child, demonstrating what will happen following compliance and noncompliance. During these dramatic reenactments, we often get a sense that the young child has internalized expectations, even if they are not always able to act on these expectations. I am struck by how many young children are shocked by the failure of the stuffed animal to follow commands.

Often, when parents return to doing CDI following the explanation of PDI, the child's play will involve time-out. The therapist is able to coach the parent's CDI while noting how the parent's play therapy skills are helping the child work through their feelings about following commands.

Initial In-Session PDI Commands

During the initial sessions of PDI, we scaffold the parent in giving commands. First, we line feed the commands to the parent word for word to ensure they give an effective command. Then, we begin having them come up with their own commands but remain ready to correct them if necessary to ensure the command is effective.

Play Commands

The initial in-session PDI commands are referred to as "play commands" in the PCIT literature (Eyberg & Funderburk, 2011; Eyberg & Matarazzo, 1980; Hembree-Kigin & McNeil, 1995; McNeil & Hembree-Kigin, 2010; Urquiza et al., 2012). However, commands involving the child's play are difficult commands for most children to follow. Imagine you are coloring a picture and someone tells you to draw a star on your picture. It is messing with your creative process. Commands to give your parent something you're playing with (taking turns) or to give your parent some of your toys (sharing) are also difficult commands for young children. So, we try to start with a command that involves briefly interrupting the child's play to hand the parent a toy they aren't currently playing with. I also have parents use nonverbal gestures such as pointing to ensure the child understands the command. For example, the parent can point to a toy and then point to their hand when they give a command for their child to hand them something.

Parents and therapists are often surprised at how willing young children are to follow these simple commands in this initial PDI session. It is a beautiful example of the power of scaffolding. By setting children up for success, we often find there is more capacity for following commands than we anticipated.

Real Commands

Real commands refer to commands to manage the child's behavior by teaching them new ways of responding in the moment or commands associated with daily living (e.g., brushing their teeth). There are often opportunities to give commands during sessions to address behavior problems. For example, the child might stand on a chair, take off their coat and whip it around their head, or grab something away from the parent. These are excellent opportunities to coach parents through how to use commands to address behavior problems. In the moment, all parents can think of is to tell their child what not to do—for example, "Don't stand on the chair." When a parent is able to give their child an effective command such as "Please get off the chair" or "Please sit in the chair," they are able to see the potential for addressing their child's behavior problems through the use of effective commands. It is also possible for the child to practice real commands associated with daily living during the session. For example, the parent can bring a toothbrush and toothpaste and have the child practice brushing their teeth during the session.

In-Session Balance Between PDI and CDI

If the child follows the command either within 5 seconds or after the warning, the parent praises the child and then returns to doing CDI for another minute or two. There is a rhythm to PDI sessions. The parent follows the child's lead, gives a command, the child complies, and the parent goes back to following the child's lead. I view this rhythm as similar to the rupture and repair we see in secure attachment relationships. There may be a brief rupture in the relationship associated with the child's misbehavior or noncompliance. However, this rupture is followed by the repair of CDI. When coaching parents during PDI, I emphasize the importance of CDI in maintaining a healthy attachment relationship while recognizing the role of limit-setting in the relationship.

Tracking Progress in PDI

We continue to track progress during PDI by spending a few minutes on assessment at the beginning of each PDI session. We continue to use parent ratings of disruptive behavior [either the ECBI (Eyberg & Pincus, 1999) or the WACB-N (Forte, Boys, & Timmer, 2012)], review of homework, and observation of parent–child interactions at the beginning of the session. We continue to observe the dyad's CDI for 5 minutes. In addition, we observe the dyad's PDI for 5 minutes.

PDI Rollout

For PDI to be successful in the long term, it is important that it be rolled out gradually at home, building on previous successes. PDI can also be rolled back, going back to a previous stage if the parent and child are struggling with the current stage.

Once parents become adept at giving effective commands, commands can provide another avenue for co-regulation. Once the child is consistently following commands, the parent can give the child a command in situations where the child is beginning to become upset. For example, if a child becomes frustrated with not being able to find a missing lego for their project, the parent can teach the child to take a break by giving the child a specific command such as "Please stand up," "Please do three jumping jacks," or "Please hand me a blue block." The child and parent learn that frustration does not inevitably lead to a meltdown. It is reassuring to both parent and child to know there is an off-ramp.

Part of the art of the PDI rollout is knowing how to gradually introduce commands in more stressful and challenging situations. It works best if the parent can begin to introduce real commands when they are relatively relaxed and calm. For example, getting ready for school and work is often a stressful time when parents feel rushed and children dig in their heels. So, once the parent decides to tackle giving commands in the morning, the parent can plan ahead and get up 30 minutes earlier than usual.

The Bottom Line

Setting limits and teaching children to follow directions is an important aspect of healthy attachment. The focus in PDI is providing parents with consistent and predictable strategies that make it easier for the child to learn to follow directions and accept their parent's limits. Clear directions from the parent and predictable consequences for noncompliance help the child learn to regulate the big emotions that come with learning to follow directions. Similarly, by providing in-the-moment clear directions to the parent, the therapist helps the parent regulate the big emotions that come with setting limits.

References

Ainsworth, M. (1967). *Infancy in Uganda*. Johns Hopkins Press.
Ainsworth, M., Blehar, M., Waters, E., & Wall, S. (1978). *Patterns of attachment: A psychological study of the strange situation*. Erlbaum.
Baumrind, D. (1966). Effects of authoritative parental control on child behavior. *Child Development, 37*(4), 887–907.
Berger, S., Adolph, K., & Lobo, S. (2005). Out of the toolbox: Toddlers differentiate wobbly and wooden handrails. *Child Development, 76*(6), 1294–1307.
Bowlby, J. (1969). *Attachment and loss. Vol 1: Attachment*. Basic Books.
Eyberg, S., & Funderburk, B. (2011). *Parent-Child Interaction Therapy Protocol*. PCIT International, Inc.
Eyberg, S., & Matarazzo, R. (1980). Training parents as therapists: A comparison between individual parent-child interaction training and parent group didactic training. *Journal of Clinical Psychology, 36*, 492–499.
Eyberg, S., & Pincus, D. (1999). *Eyberg child behavior inventory and sutter-eyberg student behavior inventory - revised*. Psychological Assessment Resources.
Forte, L., Boys, D., & Timmer, S. (2012). *The use of child behavior assessments for weekly check-ins in PCIT: WACB-N and WACB-P*. Paper presented at the 12th Annual PCIT Conference for Traumatized Children.
George, C., Kaplan, N., & Main, M. (1984). *Adult attachment interview*. University of California.
Hembree-Kigin, T., & McNeil, C. (1995). *Parent-child interaction therapy*. Plenum Press.
Kochanska, G. (2002). Committed compliance, moral self, and internalization: A mediational model. *Developmental Psychology, 38*(3), 339–351.
Main, M. (2000). The organized categories of infant, child, and adult attachment: Flexible Vs. inflexible attention under attachment-related stress. *Journal of the American Psychoanalytic Association, 48*(4), 1055–1096.
McNeil, C., & Hembree-Kigin, T. (2010). *Parent-child interaction therapy* (2nd ed.). Springer.
Powell, B., Cooper, G., Hoffman, K., & Marvin, R. (2014). *The circle of security intervention: Enhancing attachment in early parent-child relationships*. The Guilford Press.
Steele, H., & Steele, M. (2005). Understanding and resolving emotional conflict: The London parent-child project. In K. Grossman, K. Grossman, & E. Waters (Eds.), *Attachment from infancy to adulthood: The major longitudinal studies*. The Guilford Press.
Urquiza, A., Zebell, N., Timmer, S., & McGrath, J. (2012). *Course of treatment manual for PCIT-TC*. University of California Davis.
Van Zeijl, J., Mesman, J., Van Ijzendoorn, M., Bakermans-Kranenburg, M. J., Juffer, F., Stolk, M., ... Alink, L. (2006). Attachment-based intervention for enhancing sensitive discipline in mothers of 1- to 3-year-old children at risk for externalizing behavior problems: A randomized controlled trial. *Journal of Consulting and Clinical Psychology, 74*(6), 994–1005.

Chapter 6
How to Tailor Parent Coaching: Four Examples

This chapter provides fictionalized accounts of four different children with similar presenting problems but with different patterns of attachment with their parent. This chapter illustrates how the pattern of attachment influences response to intervention. It illustrates how the experience of providing the same intervention is influenced by the pattern of attachment. It describes how to tailor the intervention to better meet the child's and parent's attachment needs. These vignettes introduce concepts covered in more detail in later chapters.

Tailoring and Adaptations of Traditional PCIT

According to Sheila Eyberg, developer of Parent–Child Interaction Therapy (PCIT), "PCIT is by definition tailored to the individual family in treatment, both in process and content" (Eyberg, 2005). In addition, therapists have adapted PCIT for specific populations based on research and clinical experience with these populations (Capous et al., 2016; Timmer et al., 2006; Urquiza & McNeil, 1996; Urquiza et al., 2012). A recent study of PCIT therapists in New Zealand and Australia found that 38% of PCIT therapists reported adapting or tailoring the content. Of the therapists who adapted the protocol, 69% added content or material and 45% left out content (Woodfield et al., 2021). The most common additions to the content were helping families identify and validate their child's feelings (Woodfield et al., 2021), additions that are clearly consistent with attachment theory. The content that was most often removed was information related to the use of time-out (Woodfield et al., 2021). Therapists who left out information about the use of time-out often cited concerns about using time-out with children who were traumatized or had attachment difficulties (Woodfield et al., 2021).

© The Author(s), under exclusive license to Springer Nature Switzerland AG 2022
B. Troutman, *Attachment-Informed Parent Coaching*,
https://doi.org/10.1007/978-3-030-98570-7_6

Why to Tailor IoWA-PCIT to Working Models of Attachment

As noted in the chapter on the development of Integration of Working Models of Attachment into Parent–Child Interaction Therapy (IoWA-PCIT) (Chap. 2), adaptations I made to the traditional PCIT protocol were designed to make it more consistent with attachment theory. In addition, one of the ways I tailored parent coaching to the families I coached was to consider their working models of attachment in my coaching. Tailoring parent coaching to the child's and parents' working model of attachment is a core component of IoWA-PCIT.

If everyone's pattern of attachment was the same, this would be a much shorter book. It would make parent coaching easier but also less interesting, and it would also make this a much less interesting and diverse world. In the remaining "how to" chapters, I use research and clinical examples to explain how to understand, empathize with, and coach children and parents with different patterns of attachment. The premise of these chapters is that a truly attachment-informed approach involves understanding how the working models of attachment we bring to relationships inform our response to the world. Nowhere is this more evident than in the variety of ways in which children and their parents respond to an intervention aimed at *changing* their pattern of interaction.

In this chapter, I illustrate the different ways in which children and parents might respond to parent coaching through four fictional vignettes of children referred for help with a common early-childhood problem—oppositional behavior. The four vignettes, fictional accounts illustrating how different dyads might respond to IoWA-PCIT, provide an overview of the four primary working models identified in the research on attachment theory (Ainsworth et al., 1978; Cassidy & Marvin, 1992; George et al., 1984; Main, 2000a, 2000b; Main & Solomon, 1990).

The majority of children referred to me for IoWA-PCIT over the past decade have presented with oppositional behavior (e.g., not following directions). Although oppositional behavior evokes a particular picture of the parent and child for most therapists, I have been struck by how this same presenting problem looks different depending on the dyad and parents' attachment needs and strategies. These differences in attachment influence the child's response to this intervention, and since the intervention is delivered by coaching parents, the parent's working model of attachment influences how they interpret my statements and their response to parent coaching.

In the fictional vignettes presented in this chapter, I illustrate how four children with the same presenting problem (oppositional behavior) respond differently to the same intervention (IoWA-PCIT). I describe how the "same" intervention looks somewhat different with each family. I give examples of how the therapist needs to take the attachment needs and unique circumstances of the parent and child into account when providing the intervention.

Just as there is a myriad of different ways to get attachment needs met, there is often a myriad of different attachment relationships in the life of a child. However, all of the children in this chapter are viewed through the lens of their relationship with only one of their parents.

Example # 1: Isabella

Isabella's mother sought treatment for Isabella due to her oppositional behavior at home and school and her irritable mood. Most concerning to Isabella's mother was the way in which Isabella would look her directly in the eye while doing something her mother had told her not to do. When Isabella's mother reached out to friends to discuss her concerns, one of her friends reported having a similar problem with her daughter when she was younger. This friend indicated they had worked with a therapist who provided parent coaching using the IoWA-PCIT model and found it extremely helpful.

Isabella's mother was eager to find ways to help her daughter and trusted the therapist to help her do this. The therapist described the Child-Directed Interaction (CDI) skills that would be the focus of the first phase of treatment. She noted that the focus of CDI was child-led play. The purpose of this phase of treatment was facilitating a more positive parent–child interaction, improving Isabella's mood and regulation, and helping Isabella feel heard and understood. As a result of this experience, she was confident Isabella would become more cooperative and less oppositional. The therapist reviewed the specific skills she would be teaching Isabella's mother in CDI: labeled praise, reflection, imitation, and description. She noted that these skills were specifically designed to help her enjoy spending time with Isabella. Isabella's mother teared up a little when the therapist noted that it was sometimes difficult for mothers to enjoy spending time with their children when they were openly defiant. The therapist also described the specific types of verbalizations she would ask her to avoid during CDI—criticism, commands, and questions. Isabella's mother questioned why she was not supposed to ask questions during CDI. She accepted the therapist's explanation that answering questions can make the play less child-led and said she was willing to try this new way of interacting with her daughter.

Isabella clearly enjoyed CDI with her mother. Her mother enjoyed CDI with Isabella and saw the positive impact the skills had on her daughter and their relationship. Isabella's mother reported improvement in Isabella's mood and behavior within a couple of weeks of beginning CDI. Mother and daughter enjoyed practicing CDI for 5 minutes a day at home and CDI quickly became a part of their regular routine. Isabella's mother noted that Isabella had even begun using labeled praise with her baby brother! Isabella's mother mastered CDI in six sessions and the dyad transitioned to Parent-Directed Interaction (PDI) where the focus shifts to setting limits and increasing the child's compliance with commands. At the initial PDI session, Isabella failed to follow the first command resulting in a time-out. She followed subsequent commands and was clearly proud of her new skill in following directions, sometimes hugging her mother after she had complied with a command and reminding her mother that now they could play some more. As Isabella became more adept at following directions, she wanted to show off this skill to other important adults in her life, asking her mother if her auntie could watch her "listening practice."

Isabella and her mother are an example of the "ordinary magic" that occurs when doing attachment-informed parent coaching with a dyad where both the parent and child have secure working models of attachment. Both the parent and child are expecting to be helped by the intervention, highly motivated to improve their interaction, and lack the type of defensiveness that might interfere with treatment. Depending on treatment setting, families with secure attachment may constitute a minority or majority of the families you see. Sometimes, therapists wonder whether families with a secure attachment need intervention at all since secure attachment is a protective factor. It's important to remember that having a secure attachment does not mean a lack of struggles or problems—it means the ability to adapt and address those struggles.

Example #2: John

John's father sought treatment for John due to his oppositional behavior at home and school and his irritable mood. Although John's presenting problem is similar to Isabella's, his father's experience with seeking help was quite different. When John's father reached out to his family to discuss his concerns, they criticized the way in which he began coddling John after John's mother died. They recommended John's father spank John when he did not listen and when he got in trouble at school. John's noncompliance at school led to an evaluation by the school psychologist where John talked about being spanked by his father. When the school psychologist talked with John's father about the results of John's evaluation, she expressed concerns about the spanking. She also suggested that spanking John was likely contributing to John's misbehavior and irritability. She told John's father that she was a mandatory reporter and would need to report any spanking that left marks on John. She recommended that John's father learn better parenting skills and gave him a list of therapists that included a therapist who provided IoWA-PCIT.

Not surprisingly, John's father started treatment with a chip on his shoulder. When told treatment would begin with an observation of him and John, he immediately became defensive. He lashed out at the therapist, saying he knew other "so-called parenting experts" without children who had the "perfect answers" about how to parent. The therapist understood that John's father assumed the therapist would be another in a long line of individuals criticizing his parenting—either for being too lenient or being too harsh. She also understood that he was dealing with his own grief at the death of his wife, the unfairness of having to parent on his own, and the lack of support from others in his social network.

The therapist told John's father that the purpose of the evaluation was to help her better understand the relationship between John and his father so she could see whether IoWA-PCIT was an approach that would be useful to them. During the initial evaluation, the therapist looked carefully for positive aspects of the relationship between John and his father so she could begin giving them positive feedback. Following the initial evaluation, she told John and his father how impressed she was with John's ability to build with legos and his good manners. She failed to mention the more negative aspects of their interactions such as the father's frequent criticism of John and John's failure to follow the majority of his father's directions.

At the engage and teach session, when the therapist met with John's father alone, she spoke to the father's concerns about John and his hope for John to be more successful in school. She acknowledged the tough spot the father found himself in—trying to please family members who thought he needed to spank John more frequently and the school psychologist who had told him not to spank John. She deftly avoided the spanking controversy by simply saying she thought she could teach John's father some strategies for addressing his problems that would reduce the need to spank John. She told John's father that John had followed his directions 10% of the time during the initial evaluation and that by the end of treatment he would be following directions at least 80% of the time. She emphasized that getting to this level of compliance would take a lot of work on the part of John's father but she knew how important it was to him that his son do well in school.

When the therapist introduced the Child-Directed Interaction (CDI) skills to John's father, John's father said that he did not approve of praising children for behaviors that were expected of them. John's father also objected to not criticizing John during CDI. He said, "I've seen children who were raised without discipline and it's not pretty." The therapist agreed that criticism was a necessary part of parenting and noted that not criticizing John was only when he was doing CDI with him. The therapist told John's father that when they got to the second phase of the intervention, the Parent-Directed Interaction (PDI) or discipline phase, he would realize that the therapist believed very firmly in the importance of discipline.

In the 3 minutes prior to the initial CDI coaching session with John and his father, the therapist tried to focus on what she liked about John and his father. She remembered that John and his father were fiery, oppositional, and funny. Although most of their interactions were somewhat distant and awkward, she remembered a moment when John enjoyed entertaining his father by having the lego figures act out different scenarios. John's father initially chuckled at John's "skits" but then moved into educating him.

During the CDI coaching, the therapist saw a few moments like this and was able to chuckle along with John's father, commenting on John's creativity. As the therapist praised John's father, she noticed that John's father began to become more relaxed. However, he continued to argue with the therapist—looking toward the one-way mirror as he did so. The therapist ignored the arguing and continued to focus on what the father was doing well in interactions with his son.

The therapist began to notice changes in John during the sessions. He seemed less angry and was excited to see the therapist and play with his father. A new pattern to the CDI sessions with John and his father began to emerge. In the waiting room and in the long walk to the treatment room, the therapist saw the well-established pattern of coercive interaction between John and his father. John's father criticized the way John ran down the hall toward the room, John criticized his father's new haircut, and the therapist struggled to remember the positive aspects of John and his father as she corralled them past other offices and into the treatment room. Once they entered the treatment room, John's father began complaining about John's behavior problems at home and questioned whether therapy was making any difference. The therapist reassured John's father (and herself) that the process of changing patterns of interaction required practice and that she would continue to support John and him as they found better ways of being together during sessions.

The therapist noticed that as she was having this discussion with John's father, John had begun quietly building with the legos. The therapist commented on his lego project and how much she had enjoyed John's skits the previous week. John's father chuckled and said, "He is pretty creative when he isn't being a pain in the ass." The therapist made a mental note to focus on shaping the father's praise so it didn't end with a criticism but decided the father's half-hearted agreement with her was a step in the right direction. The therapist continued to focus her CDI coaching on validating the father's concern about his son's behavior while making observations about positive behaviors John was exhibiting during the session. Over time, as John's father soaked up the praise about himself and his son, he became softer and more positive in his interactions with her and his son.

John and his father are an example of the challenges faced when providing treatment when the child and parent have an avoidant/dismissing working model of attachment. Both the parent and child are expecting criticism and lack of emotional support from attachment figures. The therapist must understand this worldview when working with the parent and child. The parent needs the emotional experience of being nurtured, supported, and praised by the therapist in order to provide this experience to the child. Chapter 11 provides more details on working with dyads with avoidant attachment and Chap. 12 provides more details on working with parents with dismissing attachment state of mind.

Example #3: Rhonda

Rhonda's mother sought treatment for Rhonda due to her oppositional behavior at home and school and her irritable mood. Rhonda was extremely anxious about being separated from her mother. When her mother went to the bathroom, Rhonda would stand outside the door, pounding on the door and asking her when she would be out. Drop-offs at school were usually a difficult scene with the teacher and principal needing to help separate Rhonda from her mother at the door to the school. Despite Rhonda's intense anxiety at being separated from her mother, the time they spent together was characterized by constant conflict. At times, this conflict escalated to the point where Rhonda hit her mother. Rhonda's mother called her own mother several times a day to describe Rhonda's difficult behavior and seek advice about how to manage it. These phone conversations often ended in arguments about the best way to manage Rhonda's behavior. Rhonda's mother also sought advice from her therapist, and her therapy sessions increasingly revolved around discussions about Rhonda's behavior and the increasing stress it caused her mother.

Example #3: Rhonda

Rhonda's mother started IoWA-PCIT eager to talk with the therapist about problems in her relationship with Rhonda. Rhonda's mother noted that she, herself, had struggled with anxiety since she was a child and understood how difficult it was for Rhonda to control her behavior. She also talked about how her therapist thought she had post-traumatic stress disorder (PTSD) from being hit by Rhonda. Rhonda's mother expressed some concern that Rhonda would be perfectly behaved during the evaluation session when she and her daughter were observed by the therapist. Rhonda's mother talked about how her mother thought she needed to do a better job of setting limits with Rhonda but she was unable to set limits due to her PTSD. She enlisted the therapist's agreement with this statement stating, "Don't you agree that my mother should be less critical of me and more understanding about my PTSD?"

At the engage and teach session with Rhonda's mother, the therapist shared her observations of Rhonda's significant separation anxiety, behavior problems, and the frequent arguments between Rhonda and her mother. She also spoke about the moments of competence she had observed. She noted how Rhonda had moments of playing independently. She also noted how when Rhonda started to climb from the chair to the table her mother told her to get down and Rhonda followed her mother's direction. Rhonda's mother resisted the therapist's efforts to note her competence, stating, "You're the only one who thinks I can get Rhonda to listen. Just yesterday, the principal told me I really need to get her behavior under control."

In the 3 minutes prior to the first CDI coaching session with Rhonda and her mother, the therapist visualized the moment of competence she had seen. She also reminded herself to look for these moments of competence during this first session. When she entered the waiting room, Rhonda was happy to see her. She jumped up from the floor where she had been playing and ran toward the therapist. Rhonda's mother turned to Rhonda and said, "Well I guess you like her more than you like me."

Rhonda and her mother are an example of the challenges faced when providing treatment when there is a parent with a preoccupied state of mind and an ambivalent/resistant parent–child attachment relationship. Both the parent and child expect to get their attachment needs met through maintaining a conflictual relationship with attachment figures. They expect they must give up their own needs, wishes, and desires in order to be in a relationship. They also expect that if they are competent, they will lose the support of their attachment figure. The therapist must understand the worldview of the parent and child in order to effectively deliver services. The parent needs the emotional experience of having her competence recognized and acknowledged in order to recognize her child's competence. Chapter 9 provides more details on working with ambivalent/resistant dyads and Chap. 10 provides more details on working with parents with preoccupied attachment.

Example #4: Hank

Hank's mother sought treatment for Hank due to his oppositional behavior at home and school and his irritable mood. Hank's mother had recently left Hank's father due to an incident of domestic violence where the neighbors had called the police. She, Hank, and Hank's little sister were living in an apartment. Hank's mother worried that Hank's yelling at her would result in another visit from the police. Hank's mother entered treatment feeling overwhelmed by the challenges of living on her own and caring for her two children. The therapist felt a sense of urgency to address Hank's behavior in order to prevent future crises for the family.

Hank's mother brought both children to the initial evaluation for IoWA-PCIT. Hank's mother stated that she had been unable to find anyone to care for Hank's little sister during the evaluation. Faced with this dilemma, the therapist decided to go ahead with the observation. She found a dollhouse and dolls for the sister to play with in the observation room while she observed Hank and his mother's relationship. During the interaction observed by the therapist, Hank clearly seemed to be in charge. He told his mother where to sit and what to play with, and he became angry when his mother gave him commands.

During the engage and teach session, the therapist helped Hank's mother problem-solve how to have appointments without the little sister coming along. Hank's mother had recently enrolled the little sister in preschool for 3 days a week and agreed to schedule appointments for a day when the sister was in preschool. The therapist asked Hank's mother about her support system and was pleased to find that she had recently begun seeing an individual therapist.

Hank's mother arrived for the initial CDI session with Hank looking exhausted and overwhelmed. At the beginning of the session, the therapist stayed in the room with Hank and his mother for a few minutes, alternating between chatting with Hank's mother and doing CDI with Hank. At first, during the session, Hank ignored the therapist's positive descriptions of his play. However, after a couple of minutes, he warmed up and began pointing out his positive behavior to the therapist, for example, saying "I'm being careful with your toys." Hank's mother seemed surprised by this initially but began following up on Hank's comments—for example, saying, "You are being careful with the toys." Once Hank and his mother were in a calmer state of mind, the therapist transitioned to coaching Hank's mother from behind the mirror.

Hank and his mother continued in CDI for several months. The progress was slow when compared to other dyads. However, the therapist focused on the progress she saw in Hank and his mother: the decrease in Hank's bossiness toward his mother, the decrease in anxiety at spending time together, and how much they enjoyed doing CDI together.

The therapist made a gradual transition to PDI, knowing that this phase of treatment would be especially stressful for Hank and his mother. First, she introduced commands by having Hank's mother give Hank a few effective commands each session, such as, "Please hand me the blue lego." The therapist coached Hank's mother to praise Hank for complying with these commands but to ignore his noncompliance. The therapist was pleased to see that Hank followed about half of these commands. This was a considerable improvement over the initial evaluation, when Hank's mother was the only one following commands. Hank's mother became more confident and less fearful about giving commands as she saw how much her praise meant to her son. Over the next few sessions, the therapist introduced consequences for noncompliance, giving Hank and his mother ample opportunity to practice these new skills before having them try PDI at home.

Hank and his mother are an example of the challenges faced when providing treatment when there is a parent with an unresolved state of mind and a disorganized/controlling child–parent attachment relationship. There is a sense of urgency to address the problems as well as a pervasive sense of anxiety. It's important to remember that anxiety is contagious. It is easy for therapists to get caught up in the disorganized spiral. Depending on the therapist's own ways of handling anxiety, they may respond to working with unresolved attachment by becoming controlling or dysregulated themselves. Chapter 13 provides more details on working with disorganized and controlling dyads. Chapter 14 provides more details on working with parents with unresolved state of mind.

The next eight chapters provide more background and details on tailoring IoWA-PCIT to the dyad's and parent's working model of attachment. These chapters are based on the four primary working models of attachment described in the attachment literature (Ainsworth et al., 1978; George et al., 1984; Main, 2000a, 2000b; Main & Solomon, 1990). For each of the four primary working models of attachment, there is a chapter describing how to tailor coaching to the dyad's pattern of attachment (e.g., avoidant) and the parent's working model of attachment (e.g., dismissing). The reason for focusing first on the dyad and then on the parent is to help you think about both the child's attachment needs and the parent's attachment needs when tailoring the intervention.

The Bottom Line

There is a myriad of different ways to get attachment needs met for adults and children. This chapter illustrates the four most common patterns of attachment. The goal is to give therapists an idea of the need to deliver IoWA-PCIT in a manner that acknowledges differences in attachment and supports both the parent and child in more healthy relationships. Subsequent chapters will go into more detail about these patterns of attachment. My goal is to give therapists a way to understand how the pattern of interaction between the child and parent may have developed and why it may have been adaptive. In my experience, this knowledge is useful in establishing a working alliance with the parent and child.

References

Ainsworth, M., Blehar, M., Waters, E., & Wall, S. (1978). *Patterns of attachment: A psychological study of the strange situation*. Erlbaum.

Capous, D., Wallace, N., McNeil, D., & Cargo, T. (2016). Parent-child interaction therapy across diverse cultural groups. In K. Alvarez (Ed.), *Parent-child interactions and relationships: Perceptions, practices, and developmental outcomes*. Nova Publishers.

Cassidy, J., & Marvin, R. (1992). *Attachment organization in preschool children: Procedures and coding manual*. University of Virginia.

Eyberg, S. (2005). Tailoring and adapting parent-child interaction therapy to new populations. *Education and Treatment of Children, 28*(2), 197–201.

George, C., Kaplan, N., & Main, M. (1984). *Adult attachment interview*. University of California.

Main, M. (2000a). Disorganized infant, child, and adult attachment: Collapse in behavioral and attentional strategies. *Journal of the American Psychoanalytic Association, 48*, 1097–1127.

Main, M. (2000b). The organized categories of infant, child, and adult attachment: Flexible vs. inflexible attention under attachment-related stress. *Journal of the American Psychoanalytic Association, 48*, 1055–1096.

Main, M., & Solomon, J. (1990). Procedures for identifying infants as disorganized/disoriented during the Ainsworth Strange situation. In M. Greenberg, D. Cicchetti, & E. Cummings (Eds.), *Attachment in the preschool years: Theory, research, and intervention*. The University of Chicago Press.

Timmer, S., Urquiza, A., Herschell, A., McGrath, J., Zebell, N., Porter, A., & Vargas, E. (2006). Parent-child interaction therapy: Application of an empirically supported treatment to maltreated children in foster care. *Child Welfare: Journal of Policy, Practice, and Program, 85*(6), 919–939.

Urquiza, A., & McNeil, C. (1996). Parent-child interaction therapy: An intensive dyadic intervention for physically abusive families. *Child Maltreatment, 1*(2), 134–144.

Urquiza, A., Zebell, N., Timmer, S., & McGrath, J. (2012). *Course of treatment manual for PCIT-TC*. University of California Davis.

Woodfield, M., Cargo, T., Merry, S., & Hetrick, S. (2021). Barriers to clinician implementation of parent-child interaction therapy (PCIT) in New Zealand and Australia: What role for time-out? *International Journal of Environmental Research and Public Health, 18*, 13116.

Chapter 7
Ordinary Magic: How to Tailor Coaching for Dyads with Secure Attachment

This chapter describes the characteristics of a secure child–parent attachment relationship. I describe the foundation of a secure attachment relationship—the variety of ways infants and young children signal their attachment needs and the characteristics of the sensitively responsive caregiving associated with the development of secure attachment. I discuss how secure attachment may be adaptive and the prevalence of secure attachment. I describe how parent coaching can promote secure attachment and the course of IoWA-PCIT with secure dyads.

Each child's path to a strategy for getting their attachment needs met is unique. And the way they get their attachment needs met is unique with each parent, that is, young children develop a different pattern of attachment with each primary caregiver. So, it is possible for a child to have a secure relationship with one parent and an insecure relationship with another parent. While we would hope for every child to have a secure attachment relationship with each parent, research suggests that having a secure attachment with at least one parent provides powerful protection (Kochanska & Kim, 2013).

How to Recognize Secure Child–Parent Attachment

The hallmark of secure attachment is clear communication. In secure child–parent attachment relationships, there is a balance between attachment and exploration. A secure attachment between a parent and child involves several key characteristics. Of course, there are changes in the relationship between parent and child across the life span, but the general characteristics of secure attachment remain consistent throughout the life span and are recognizable at each developmental stage.

First, secure attachment relationships provide what Bowlby and Ainsworth have called a haven of safety (Ainsworth et al., 1978; Bowlby, 1969). The term secure is used for this type of attachment relationship because it is the opposite of feeling anxious. Having a secure attachment relationship provides a sense of safety and security. A haven of safety is the equivalent of a den for mammals like foxes and wolves. That is, it is the safe place the child can, does, and wants to go to whenever they are distressed. Second, secure attachment relationships provide what Bowlby and Ainsworth called a secure base (Ainsworth et al., 1978; Bowlby, 1969). The secure base is a strong tether that allows children to go out and explore their world, knowing that the parent has their back if they run into difficulties. In secure attachment relationships, there is a balance for the child between feeling free to go out and explore and feeling free to come back to the parent for comfort when distressed—a balance between exploration and attachment, or what more poetic types might call the balance between work and love. Finding that balance is the work of a lifetime for each of us, but it begins in infancy.

Secure attachment is characterized by clear communication of attachment needs. Initially, infants primarily communicate their attachment needs with crying (Ainsworth, 1967, 1969; Ainsworth et al., 1978). The baby's developmental achievements allow them new ways to communicate their attachment needs to their parents. For example, once babies begin to smile, they communicate their attachment needs through smiling and the development of their locomotor skills allows them to communicate their attachment needs with behaviors such as reaching for their parent and following their parent.

Preschool-aged children have a larger repertoire of ways in which to clearly communicate their attachment needs (Cassidy & Marvin, 1992; Moss et al., 2004; 2015). In addition to communicating through crying and behavior, preschool-aged children communicate their attachment needs through language. Preschool-aged children talk with parents about their feelings—verbally expressing both displeasure and excitement. Preschool-aged children also begin to use play to express their perspectives on attachment relationships—hugging their baby dolls, putting their baby dolls to bed, and scolding their baby dolls in ways that reflect their experiences with attachment relationships.

How to Recognize Secure Attachment in Infant Strange Situation Procedure

After thousands of hours observing infants in their homes in Uganda and Baltimore, Maryland, Mary Ainsworth and her colleagues developed the Strange Situation Procedure to demonstrate the balance between the attachment system and the exploratory system in babies (Ainsworth, 1967; Ainsworth et al., 1978). The Strange Situation Procedure was designed to activate both the exploratory system and the attachment system through a series of brief situations. The parent and child enter a room with toys (3 minutes), a stranger enters the room (3 minutes), the parent leaves the child with the stranger (3 minutes or less if the child is unduly distressed), the parent reunites with the child (3 minutes), the parent leaves the infant in the room alone (3 minutes or less if the child is unduly distressed), the stranger enters the room (3 minutes or less if the child is unduly distressed), and the parent returns and reunites with the child (3 minutes).

I never tire of watching the mini drama of separation and reunion play out during the 21-minute Strange Situation Procedure.

Let me take you through a Strange Situation Procedure with a securely attached infant and her mother. First, the mother and baby enter a room with toys, a situation designed to activate the infant's exploratory system. In the Strange Situation Procedure, these moments of exploration often involve brief looks back at the parent to ensure that it is safe to explore. Then, the infant's attachment system is activated by having the parent briefly leave the room and leave the baby with a stranger. During the separation, securely attached infants often interact with the stranger while indicating they are missing the parent, for example, by vocalizing to the stranger and pointing at the door. During the reunions with the parent, securely attached babies engage in behaviors to rebalance the attachment–exploration balance. Some securely attached babies crawl or walk to the door, then sit or stand at the door and cry, waiting for their parent's return. When the parent returns, the infant reaches for the parent to be picked up. The power of what we call co-regulation is obvious in this moment, when the infant calms quickly and wants to begin exploring again. Not all securely attached infants become distressed during the separation. Some securely attached babies wait quietly for their parent's return, smile, and greet the parent when they return and then return to smooth, enjoyable interactions with their parent.

Comparison of Strange Situation Procedure in Infants and Preschool-Aged Children

After years of seeing babies in Strange Situation Procedures, I have marveled at how different it is to see children a mere year older in a similar paradigm (Cassidy & Marvin, 1992). What a difference language makes in relationships. Parents are able to explain to the child that they are leaving. The child is able to ask the parent why they are leaving, negotiate with the parent about leaving, and express their feelings about the separation. When the parent returns after a brief separation, the child is able to talk with the parent about what happened during the separation, tell them about their feelings about the separation, and ask the parent why they left. Although nonverbal behavior continues to be important in observations of parent–child interactions, the verbal, cognitive, and motor skills of preschool-aged children also provide rich sources of information about the relationship.

How to Recognize Secure Attachment in Preschool Strange Situation Procedure

When the parent is about to leave for a brief separation during the preschool Strange Situation Procedure, the child may try to negotiate with the parent to stay and play or may ask to go with them. As with the infant Strange Situation Procedure, the reunion—that is, when the parent returns from a brief separation—is the moment when the preschool-aged child clearly communicates their attachment needs. As with infants, they often greet the returning parent with nonverbal means such as a smile, but the smile is often accompanied by verbalizations. The child may describe what they were doing while the parent was gone—for example, "I built a tower!" The child may describe their feeling during the separation—for example, "I was lonely." The hallmark of secure attachment is the child's ability to directly express whatever they experienced during the separation, when the parent returns.

Let me take you through a preschool Strange Situation Procedure to give you a sense of a preschool-aged child with a secure attachment. Two-and-a-half-year-old Mary confidently enters the playroom with her mother. She gravitates to the blocks on the floor and begins building, occasionally looking to her mother for affirmation of her building success. After 5 minutes, her mother leaves the room and enters the observation room. Mary continues to play and build. To a casual observer, there is no real change in her demeanor during this absence of her mother. A more careful observer would note that Mary's play is somewhat less creative and joyful than when her mother is in the room. After a 5-minute absence, her mother returns to the room. Mary immediately greets her and asks her mother where she has been. Her mother responds that she was talking with the therapist and asks Mary what she did while she was gone. Mary shows her mother what she built with her blocks and begins building with the enjoyment she demonstrated prior to the separation.

Development of Secure Child–Parent Attachment

Attachment Signals

Secure attachment develops when parents are responsive to their child's attachment signals. Attachment signals are the different ways infants and young children signal that they need their parent's attention and support. In infants, the most common and most effective way of signaling a need is through crying. As infants develop, they are able to add more ways of signaling their needs. One of the ways they signal as they get a bit older is by smiling. The type of smile infants give their parents when they recognize them as someone very special to them, often referred to as a social smile, usually happens when the baby is between 4 and 6 weeks old. This first broad smile, a baby's signal that she recognizes the person or people she is attached to, is a very special milestone for her parents. Much of the literature on attachment highlights and brings into focus things we all know but have not studied, and the information about how a baby's social smile is one of the building blocks of child–parent attachment is a good example of this. Who can imagine not responding to an infant's smile by smiling back?

Another attachment signal seen early on is reaching. Infants reach out to their parents when their parents approach their crib, as a signal to be picked up. Infants also signal their attachment needs through clinging—for example, clinging to their parent when they do not want to be put down. As infants become more competent in their motor abilities, their attachment signals become more sophisticated. Once infants are able to crawl, they often crawl after a parent when the parent leaves the room. When infants are able to move, they can walk or run after a parent. The ability to walk coincides with increased separation anxiety and stranger anxiety—the latter a handy evolutionary defense against young toddlers being taken up by strangers or wandering off on their own.

Once children are able to talk, they can use language to communicate their attachment needs. They can call out to their parents in the middle of the night when they have a nightmare. They can tell their parents when they are mad, sad, angry, or happy. On the other side of the attachment–exploration balance, they can also use language to tell their parents about their explorations.

Sensitive Responsiveness to Attachment Signals

Therapists who are adept observers of a child's attachment signals can begin to look for the variety of ways in which parents respond to these signals—and the moments when they fail to respond to them. Mary Ainsworth used the term sensitive responsiveness to describe the type of response seen in parents who develop a secure infant–parent attachment relationship with their child (Ainsworth, 1967; Ainsworth et al., 1978). Sensitive responsiveness is defined as a prompt, consistent, and appropriate response to a child's attachment signal. The research on sensitive responsiveness is clear—by responding to the child's attachment signals, the parent teaches the child to learn to trust that their needs will be met and the child also learns to trust themselves (van Ijzendoorn, 1995).

The reason *prompt* responses are important is that infants and young children have fleeting attention spans and are easily frustrated. So, for a response to be sensitive to the needs of a developing child, it must be immediate. The difference between responding immediately to the cries of an infant who has awoken in a strange place and is frightened and responding after he has become extremely frightened and upset is huge.

A *consistent* response is a response that fits with the child's signal—that is, it is consistent with what the child is signaling. When a parent responds in a consistent manner to their child's attachment signal, the action can be so smooth it is easy to overlook the attachment signal. For example, I have seen parents make slight postural adjustments when holding their baby that result in the infant snuggling in closer and settling. I wasn't even aware that the infant was uncomfortable until I noticed the mother shifting the infant slightly in her arms and the baby settling. The baby communicated, "I'm uncomfortable," and the mother responded consistently by moving in a way that made the baby more comfortable.

The absence of a consistent response to a child's attachment signal is more likely to capture our attention. An example of an inconsistent response is a parent who responds to a child reaching out his arms to be picked up, by turning away. The baby reaching for the parent signals "I want to be picked up" and the parent turning away is an inconsistent response to this communication. Other examples of inconsistent responses to attachment signals are responding to a baby's distress by scolding him for crying or responding to a child's smile by scowling.

An *appropriate* response to the child's signal takes into account what the child needs. For example, the infant's crying indicates he is in distress and needs something, but it doesn't communicate what exactly he needs. A baby who is crying may need a diaper change, a cuddle, or to be fed. Figuring out the appropriate response takes a bit of detective work as well as some empathy. The parent needs to sort through the data of the baby's last diaper change and feeding. And the parent also needs to be able to put themselves in the baby's shoes and think about what the baby might be needing in this moment.

How Secure Attachment May Be Adaptive for the Child

Each of the patterns of attachment is adaptive. Each pattern allows the child to get their attachment needs met with a particular caregiver. The "ordinary magic" of secure attachment is the self-confidence that comes with knowing your parent has your back whether you are exploring or facing a situation where you need to check in with someone older and wiser (Masten, 2001). Secure attachment is adaptive because it provides the child with more options. Children in securely attached dyads are comfortable both with exploring their environment and seeking support when needed. Children in securely attached dyads are also able to directly communicate their feelings and concerns to their parents, taking some of the guesswork out of addressing the child's concerns.

Prevalence of Secure Attachment Pattern

Secure attachment is the most prevalent pattern of attachment in community samples (Greenberg et al., 1991; Kochanska & Kim, 2013; Leigh et al., 2004; Moss et al., 2004; Speltz et al., 1990; Troutman et al., 2010; van Ijzendoorn et al., 1999). More than half of child–parent dyads in community samples have a secure attachment.

Secure attachment is also the most prevalent pattern of attachment in children referred to me for IoWA-PCIT. Half of the child–parent dyads evaluated for IoWA-PCIT are securely attached.

I'll admit that I was initially surprised by the number of securely attached dyads seeking help. I expected the frequency of secure attachment in clinical populations to be much lower than it is. I have come to realize that seeking help when there are problems is part of the protection conferred by secure attachment.

As therapists, we are focused on problems. After all, that is why parents seek our assistance—because there is a problem they want to address. Because of the association of behavior problems and attachment, there is a tendency to look for problems in the relationship. I hope to reorient you to looking for solutions in the relationship—and often this means tapping into the underlying security that is already present in the relationship. I encourage you to look for security and for a secure attachment in the dyads you work with.

How to Promote Secure Attachment: Coaching Parents To Be More Sensitively Responsive to Attachment Signals

There are a number of different reasons why parents might fail to respond sensitively to their child's attachment cues. I find it helpful to think about the different stages of responding to the attachment signal of an infant or a child. This can be a useful way to scaffold parents to become more sensitively responsive to their child's attachment cues. First, the parent must perceive the attachment signal. They must notice that the infant or child is crying, smiling, reaching, walking toward them, telling them that they feel sad, or telling them this is the best day of their life. Second, the parent must identify what the infant or child needs. Third, the parent must respond in a way that acknowledges the attachment cue.

I find it helpful to think about these three stages when working with parents. I start with the first stage, pointing out the attachment signal. This has become second nature to me now, but when I first learned to do this it seemed incredibly awkward because it seemed so obvious. For example, you might say something like "He is smiling at you." Or, "She just made eye contact with you." Or, "He is really upset right now." For many parents, having an extra pair of eyes to notice their child's cues is enough for them to respond in a prompt, consistent, and appropriate manner to their child's attachment cues.

Other parents notice the child's cues either on their own or with the therapist's help but have difficulty identifying what the child needs. When working with these parents, it can be useful to lend them your detective skills. For example, you might say something like "He is really crying. I wonder whether he is hungry." Or, "She looks so excited to play with you today. I wonder if she needed some mom time." By linking the observation with guesses about the child's needs and experiences, you give the parent a model for developing their own detective skills.

Once parents perceive the attachment signal and identify what the child needs, you can begin helping them implement a prompt, consistent, and appropriate response to the child's attachment cues. Often, this is a matter of supporting their instincts in the face of previous misinformation or their own childhood attachment history. The most common example is parents who are worried they will spoil their baby by responding to their cries. For example, you might say, "Your dad instincts were right on target. He just wanted to be held." Or, "I can see how hard it is for you to sit back and let him explore. Great job of letting him solve this problem on his own."

Promoting secure attachment is a bit easier with secure dyads since in those cases we primarily need to reinforce what is already working. However, don't underestimate the importance of your role in reinforcing the security of the attachment relationship. Parents are bombarded with advice about child-rearing these days, especially if their child has some struggles with emotional and behavioral regulation. We have an important role in pointing out what is already working in their relationship with their child.

How to Promote Secure Attachment in Infants

Studies on interventions during the first year of life indicate that relatively minor changes in the parent's caregiving can promote secure attachment. One of my favorite intervention studies is an early study where mothers were given either a soft baby carrier (Snuggli) or a plastic infant seat following their infant's birth and asked to use it with their child every day (Anisfeld et al., 1990). The rate of secure attachment among mothers given a Snuggli (83%) was more than twice the rate among mothers given a plastic infant seat (38%) (Anisfeld et al., 1990).

I find it fascinating that this seemingly simple intervention yielded such a large impact on the security of the infant–parent relationship. I'm especially interested in this because I know that plastic infant seats are not inherently incompatible with secure attachment. During in-home visits, I have observed attuned mothers who were adept at reading their infant's attachment signals while their child was in a plastic infant seat—for example, putting the child's infant seat across from them while they folded clothes so they, the mother, could look up and vocalize to the child while folding clothes. Beatrice Beebe's research on early interactions associated with attachment (Beebe et al., 2010; Beebe & Lachmann, 2014) was able to determine the differences between dyads that would become secure and those that would become insecure when infants were sitting in a plastic infant seat. The dyads who exhibited secure attachment at 12 months were already in sync in their face-to-face interactions at 4 months (Beebe et al., 2010, 2016; Beebe & Lachmann, 2014). Mothers paused when their infants looked away and waited for the infant to return their attention, mirrored their baby's moods, and imitated their baby's movements.

I suspect the reason for the positive impact of the Snuggli is twofold: the increased positive physical contact between the mother and child, and the fact that holding the child close in the Snuggli makes it easier for the mother to attune to the child's signals. In human development, until fairly recently it was rare for infants not to be carried close to their mother's bodies. I suspect it is easier for caregivers to tap into the inborn attachment drive when the infant is physically nearby.

How to Promote Secure Attachment in Toddlers and Preschool-Aged Children

I think of Child-Directed Interaction (CDI) (described in Chap. 4) as being like a Snuggli for toddlers and preschoolers. During CDI, the child is physically close to the parent and the parent is attuned to the child in a way that facilitates the parent's inborn attachment drive.

During our coaching, we have the opportunity to promote secure attachment by pointing out the child's cues as well as the ways the parent can foster or is already fostering a healthy attachment relationship with their child. For example, we might focus on the attachment part of the attachment–exploration balance by saying, "He just needs a cuddle with mom before he is ready to play today." Or we might focus on the exploration part of the attachment–exploration balance by saying, "That toy is a bit advanced for his age. He is able to do it because of your CDI skills."

We can point out to parents the ways their child is beginning to engage in a goal-directed partnership with them. For example, "I love that he gave you the purple crayon because he remembered that purple was your favorite color." We can also point out the ways in which their child is beginning to repair when there are ruptures in the relationship. For example, "It's great that he apologized for accidentally knocking over your tower."

Course of IoWA-PCIT with Secure Dyads

Research indicates that both secure and insecure dyads demonstrate significant decreases in disruptive behavior in IoWA-PCIT (Troutman, 2016). However, as suggested above, the path to decreasing disruptive behavior seems smoother with dyads who start treatment with a secure attachment relationship. Although the title of this chapter refers to tailoring IoWA-PCIT for children with secure attachment, the truth is that the intervention requires less tailoring for children with secure attachment than for children in insecure attachment relationships with their parents. In my clinical experience, dyads with a secure attachment come into treatment with less severe disruptive behavior than dyads with an insecure attachment. In addition to having less severe problems at the beginning of treatment, both the child and parent are more likely to trust me and each other. Thus, they are less resistant to changing their pattern of interaction. They seem able to incorporate new ways of interacting without giving up their sense of who they are. They have a more flexible view of the world which can incorporate new ideas and ways of being together. Consequently, dyads with secure attachment spend less time in IoWA-PCIT. The majority of secure dyads I've seen in IoWA-PCIT demonstrate significant improvement after a few sessions, and most of them complete treatment in less than 20 sessions.

The Bottom Line

The building blocks of secure attachment are the thousands of moments where parents respond sensitively to their child's attachment cues over the course of their infancy and early childhood. For parents to respond sensitively to their child's needs for attachment and exploration, the parents must perceive the attachment cue, identify the need, and respond promptly, consistently, and appropriately. As therapists, we can scaffold parent's sensitive responsiveness to their child's attachment cues by helping them observe the cue, figure out the need, and respond sensitively.

References

Ainsworth, M. (1967). *Infancy in Uganda*. Johns Hopkins Press.
Ainsworth, M. (1969). Object relations, dependency and attachment: A theoretical review of the infant-mother relationship. *Child Development, 40*, 969–1025.
Ainsworth, M., Blehar, M., Waters, E., & Wall, S. (1978). *Patterns of attachment: A psychological study of the strange situation*. Erlbaum.
Anisfeld, A., Casper, V., Nozyce, M., & Cunningham, N. (1990). Does infant carrying promote attachment? An experimental study of the effects of increased physical contact on the development of attachment. *Child Development, 61*(5), 1617–1627.
Beebe, B., Cohen, P., & Lachmann, F. (2016). *The mother-infant interaction picture book*. Norton.
Beebe, B., Jaffe, J., Markese, S., Buck, K., Chen, H., Cohen, P., ... Feldstein, S. (2010). The origins of 12-month attachment: A microanalysis of 4-month mother-infant interaction. *Attachment & Human Development, 12*(1–2), 3–141.
Beebe, B., & Lachmann, F. (2014). *The origins of attachment: Infant research and adult treatment*. Routledge.
Bowlby, J. (1969). *Attachment and loss. Vol 1: Attachment*. Basic Books.
Cassidy, J., & Marvin, R. (1992). *Attachment organization in preschool children: Procedures and coding manual*. University of Virginia.
Greenberg, M., Speltz, M., DeKlyen, M., & Endriga, M. (1991). Attachment security in preschoolers with and without externalizing behavior problems: A replication. *Development and Psychopathology, 3*, 413–430.
Kochanska, G., & Kim, S. (2013). Early attachment organization with both parents and future behavior problems: From infancy to middle childhood. *Child Development, 84*(1), 283–296.
Leigh, I., Brice, P., & Meadow-Orlans, K. (2004). Attachment in deaf mothers and their children. *Journal of Deaf Studies and Deaf Education, 9*(2), 176–188.
Masten, A. (2001). Ordinary magic. Resilience processes in development. *American Psychologist, 56*(3), 227–238.

References

Moss, E., Cyr, C., & Dubois-Comtois, K. (2004). Attachment at early school age and developmental risk: Examining family contexts and behavior problems of controlling-caregiving, controlling-punitive, and behaviorally disorganized children. *Developmental Psychology, 40*(4), 519–532.

Moss, E., Lecompte, V., & Bureau, J. (2015). *Preschool and early school-age attachment rating scales (PARS)*. University of Quebec at Montreal.

Speltz, M., Greenberg, M., & DeKlyen, M. (1990). Attachment in preschoolers with disruptive behavior: A comparison of clinic-referred and nonproblem children. *Development and Psychopathology, 2*, 31–46.

Troutman, B. (2016). Does security of attachment moderate response to parent-child intervention for disruptive behavior? In K. Alvarez (Ed.), *Parent-child interactions and relationships: Perceptions, practice and developmental outcomes* (pp. 45–60). Nova Publishers.

Troutman, B., Arndt, S., Caspers, K. M., & Yucuis, R. (2010). *Infant negative emotionality moderates the association between quantity of nonfamilial day care and infant-mother attachment*. Paper presented at the 57th Annual Meeting of the American Academy of Child & Adolescent Psychiatry, New York, NY.

van Ijzendoorn, M. (1995). Adult attachment representations, parental responsiveness, and infant attachment: A meta-analysis on the predictive validity of the adult attachment interview. *Psychological Bulletin, 117*(3), 387–403.

van Ijzendoorn, M., Schungel, C., & Bakermans-Kranenburg, M. J. (1999). Disorganized attachment in early childhood: Meta-analysis of precursors, concomitants, and sequelae. *Development and Psychopathology, 11*, 225–249.

Chapter 8
Open to Change: How to Tailor Coaching for Parents with Secure/Autonomous Attachment

This chapter discusses how to coach parents with a secure/autonomous working model of attachment. Clues to recognizing secure attachment are discussed, including recognition of parents who are "earned secure"—that is, parents who have overcome difficult childhood experiences of their own and developed secure attachment relationships with their children.

How to Recognize Parents' Secure/Autonomous Working Model of Attachment

There are two clues to recognizing a secure/autonomous working model of attachment in parents: their communication with us and the quality of their relationship with their child. On the Adult Attachment Interview (AAI), a narrative assessment used to assess adult attachment in research studies, individuals with secure/autonomous attachment are good storytellers (George et al., 1984; Main, 2000; Steele & Steele, 2008). They are good communicators who keep the need of their audience, that is, the interviewer, in mind. They are able to give vivid descriptions of themselves and others. Because of the vividness of their description and their clear communication, some of their descriptions of their child and their own reactions can sometimes be surprising to therapists. For example, they may describe feeling angry at their young child when the child won't sleep.

Since the parent's working model of attachment is the strongest predictor of the quality of their child's relationship with them, the attachment assessment of the parent–child relationship gives us an idea of the parent's working model of attachment (van Ijzendoorn, 1995). That is, if the child–parent attachment relationship is secure, it is likely the parent has a secure/autonomous working model (van Ijzendoorn, 1995). We also can see indicators of the parent's working model by how they communicate with the child. Parents with a secure working model tend to communicate clearly with their child during the assessment—for example, telling the child they will be leaving before they leave the playroom.

How to Recognize Earned Secure Working Model of Attachment

Earned secure attachment is a classification in the adult attachment research that is especially relevant to parent coaching (Main, 2000; Steele & Steele, 2008). Individuals with an earned secure working model of attachment describe difficult childhood experiences but describe them in a way that is balanced and forgiving of their parents.

How Secure/Autonomous Attachment May Be Adaptive

Parents with secure/autonomous state of mind are considered especially good candidates for parent–child interventions. As noted by a research group examining attachment in children referred for disruptive behavior, parents with secure/autonomous attachment "are better able to learn and use the 'here-and-now' skills important to current relationships" (Greenberg et al., 1991). In other words, one of the ways in which secure/autonomous attachment is adaptive is the greater flexibility of secure parents who value attachment relationships and are open to new ideas about interacting with their child.

In a study of an attachment-based home-visiting intervention (Korfmacher et al., 1997), mothers with secure/autonomous attachment were more likely to seek assistance with parenting tasks and rarely sought crisis intervention. Thus, parents with secure/autonomous attachment are a good fit for an intervention focused on promoting positive attachment with their child and learning new ways to interact as they are open to help with parenting.

Attachment researcher Deborah Jacobvitz notes that individuals with secure/autonomous attachment "benefit more from intervention programs than do adults classified as insecure" (Jacobvitz, 2008). As with secure attachment in infants and young children, adults with secure/autonomous working models of attachment have greater flexibility, making it easier for them to make use of new ideas about how to parent their child. They value relationships—a state of mind they bring to their relationship with the therapist and their relationship with their child.

Parents with secure/autonomous attachment also value facilitating their child's growth and independence. They are comfortable with conflict and with addressing ruptures in relationships—whether those ruptures are with their child or with the therapist (Miller-Bottome et al., 2017; 2019). Not surprisingly, research on the communication of secure/autonomous patients with their therapist suggests it is easier to form a therapeutic alliance with patients who trust in relationships (Talia et al., 2014). I have found the research on how individuals with secure/autonomous attachment communicate with their therapists very helpful in understanding why it seems easier to coach secure/autonomous parents (Miller-Bottome et al., 2017, 2019; Talia et al., 2014).

As with securely attached children, adults with secure attachment use their therapist as a safe haven—seeking proximity and maintaining contact through the ways in which they communicate with their therapist (Miller-Bottome et al., 2017, 2019; Talia et al., 2014; 2015). The specific details of how securely attached patients communicate with their therapists provide a model for thinking about effective communication in therapeutic encounters. Some of the ways in which securely attached individuals seek proximity with their therapist are to ask for help, ask for advice, and ask for the therapist's opinion. For example, a parent with a secure/autonomous attachment might say, "I don't know how to get him to follow directions. He is so different than his older sister. I know he feels bad about how often we yell at him. I would really like for things to go more smoothly between the two of us. Do you have ideas of what might help?" Another way in which secure adults seek proximity with their therapist is through openly disclosing distressful events and feelings, including distressful events during the therapy. For example, a parent with a secure/autonomous attachment might say, "It was upsetting when you told me to ignore his disrespectful language toward me. I know my parent would have punished me for that language."

One of the ways in which secure adults maintain contact with their therapist is to praise the therapist and the therapy—pointing out the positive aspects of the therapist and their work together (Miller-Bottome et al., 2017, 2019; Talia et al., 2014, 2015). In Chap. 4, I noted the concern that some therapists have about the use of praise. So, I find it reassuring that praising is consistent with secure/autonomous attachment.

Securely attached individuals are also able to use the therapist as a secure base for exploring new ideas. Secure individuals are willing to challenge their therapist—asserting themselves by proposing goals for therapy and expressing concerns about the therapeutic tasks (Miller-Bottome et al., 2017, 2019; Talia et al., 2014; 2015). In addition to sharing distressing experiences, they are also open to sharing positive experiences. Secure individuals are also reflective—they are able to dig below the surface and think about alternative perspectives of their own or their child's experience.

When there is a conflict or rupture in the therapeutic relationship, patients with secure/autonomous attachment are also better at repair (Miller-Bottome et al., 2017, 2019). Ruptures in the therapeutic relationship, that is, moments when the patient feels misunderstood or not helped by the therapist, are just as likely to occur with secure/autonomous patients as they are with patients with insecure working models of attachment (Miller-Bottome et al., 2017, 2019). This is a reminder that conflict and misunderstandings are a feature of all relationships. The protective magic provided by a secure working model of attachment is the ability to communicate about these difficulties and to repair the relationship.

Prevalence of Secure/Autonomous Attachment

Secure/autonomous attachment is the most prevalent type of attachment in community samples with approximately half of adults classified as secure/autonomous on the AAI (Booth-LaForce & Roisman, 2014; Caspers et al., 2007; van Ijzendoorn, 1995). Secure/autonomous attachment is also the most prevalent type of attachment in a study of low-income mothers participating in an attachment-based home-visiting intervention (Korfmacher et al., 1997). Rates of secure/autonomous attachment are significantly lower in a study of mothers seeking treatment for their child's behavior problems (22%) (Routh et al., 1995).

Course of IoWA-PCIT with Secure/Autonomous Parents

In my clinical experience, parents with secure/autonomous attachment are able to make changes more quickly. They are open to change and reflection, so the work of changing their pattern of interaction comes easier and is less anxiety-provoking than it is for parents with insecure working models of attachment. Secure/autonomous parents are able to use our coaching to interact with their children in new ways and reflect on the experiences they bring to parenting.

When working with parents with secure/autonomous attachment, it feels easier to talk with them directly about our concerns. For example, if we notice a parent has difficulty following their child's lead in Child-Directed Interaction (CDI), we can say to them, "It looks like it's a little tough for you to let him lead the play." Parents with a secure/autonomous state of mind are likely to perceive this observation as we intended it—as an observation of their struggle. Because they tend to be open to change and reflective, they may even reflect on why it is difficult for them to follow their child's lead.

When we get to the Parent-Directed Interaction (PDI) phase of IoWA-PCIT, secure/autonomous parents are open to sharing their concerns about this phase of treatment. This allows us to talk through these concerns prior to coaching this new set of skills. I find many secure/autonomous parents also share their own experiences with being disciplined when we get to PDI and reflect on how these experiences have colored their perceptions of disciplining their child.

Course of IoWA-PCIT with Earned Secure Parents

The parents who have an earned secure working model of attachment have often had their own therapy to address their childhood attachment experiences. When they have children of their own, these individuals find themselves in a difficult position. The people that many parents turn to when they have parenting struggles, their own parents, is not a great option when they have concerns about their own childhood. So, it makes sense that they would turn to a therapist to address their concerns about their child. Parents with earned secure working models of attachment also face the additional challenge of figuring out the role their parents (their children's grandparents) and other family members will play in their children's lives. Sometimes, circumstances have changed, and grandparents are able to develop a healthy relationship with their grandchildren—a relationship that does not replicate the parents' difficult childhood. Other times, parents need to limit interactions with grandparents due to concerns about the impact these interactions may have on their child.

I often schedule parent-only sessions (i.e., sessions where the child is not present) to discuss parents' concerns about their children's interactions with grandparents or other family members. I also offer to meet with grandparents and other family members and, if the parent thinks it is appropriate, to coach grandparents in Child-Directed Interaction (CDI) (described in Chap. 4) and Parent-Directed interaction (PDI) (described in Chap. 5). These sessions can be both healing and bittersweet for parents as they watch their child have the type of relationship with their parents they yearned for as a child.

The Bottom Line

It is easier for secure parents to develop secure relationships with their children and to develop a secure therapeutic relationship with a therapist. There is no getting around the fact that this makes our job as parent coaches considerably easier. It doesn't mean there won't be conflicts and rough patches in our relationship with secure parents, but it does mean it will be easier to repair those ruptures when they occur. Because secure/autonomous parents have a relatively balanced view of relationships, they approach their relationship with us with balance—allowing us to serve as both a secure base and a safe haven. As a secure base, we are able to help parents explore new ideas for improving their relationship with their child and ways they would like to change as a parent. As a safe haven, we are able to provide support when they express concerns and difficulties in their relationship with their child.

Because parents with secure/autonomous attachment understand the importance of relationships and value attachment relationships, an approach that focuses on developing a more positive, rewarding relationship with their child makes sense to them. Since they are open to new ideas and flexible enough to incorporate them into their view of relationships, we are able to develop a collaborative relationship in our shared goal of improving their child's social-emotional development.

References

Booth-LaForce, C., & Roisman, G. (2014). The adult attachment interview: Psychometrics, stability and change from infancy and developmental origins. *Monographs of the Society for Research in Child Development, 79*(3), 1–185.

Caspers, K. M., Yucuis, R., Troutman, B., Arndt, S., & Langbehn, D. (2007). A sibling adoption study of adult attachment: The influence of shared environment on attachment state of mind. *Attachment & Human Development, 9*(4), 375–391.

George, C., Kaplan, N., & Main, M. (1984). *Adult Attachment Interview*. University of California.

Greenberg, M., Speltz, M., DeKlyen, M., & Endriga, M. (1991). Attachment security in preschoolers with and without externalizing behavior problems: A replication. *Development and Psychopathology, 3*, 413–430.

Jacobvitz, D. (2008). Afterword: Reflections on clinical applications of the adult attachment interview. In H. Steele & M. Steele (Eds.), *Clinical applications of the adult attachment interview*. The Guilford Press.

Korfmacher, J., Adam, E., Ogawa, J., & Egeland, B. (1997). Adult attachment: Implications for the therapeutic process in a home visitation intervention. *Applied Developmental Science, 1*(1), 43–52.

Main, M. (2000). The organized categories of infant, child, and adult attachment: Flexible vs. inflexible attention under attachment-related stress. *Journal of the American Psychoanalytic Association, 48*, 1055–1096.

Miller-Bottome, M., Talia, A., Eubanks, C., Safran, J., & Muran, J. (2019). Secure in-session attachment predicts rupture resolution: Negotiating a secure base. *Psychoanalytic Psychology, 36*(2), 132–138.

Miller-Bottome, M., Talia, A., Safran, J., & Muran, J. (2017). Resolving alliance ruptures from an attachment-informed perspective. *Psychoanalytic Psychology, 35*(2), 175–183.

Routh, C., Hill, J., Steele, H., Elliott, C., & Dewey, M. (1995). Maternal attachment status, psychosocial stressors and problem behaviour: Follow-up after parent training courses for conduct disorder. *Journal of Child Psychology and Psychiatry, 36*(7), 1179–1198.

Steele, H., & Steele, M. (2008). *Clinical applications of the adult attachment interview*. The Guilford Press.

Talia, A., Daniel, S., Miller-Bottome, M., Brambilla, D., Miccoli, D., Safran, J., & Lingiardi, V. (2014). AAI predicts patients' in-session interpersonal behavior and discourse: A "move to the level of the relation" for attachment-informed psychotherapy research. *Attachment & Human Development, 16*(2), 192–209.

Talia, A., Miller-Bottome, M., & Daniel, S. (2015). Assessing attachment in psychotherapy: Validation study of the patient attachment coding system. *Clinical Psychology & Psychotherapy, 24*, 149–161.

van Ijzendoorn, M. (1995). Adult attachment representations, parental responsiveness, and infant attachment: A meta-analysis on the predictive validity of the adult attachment interview. *Psychological Bulletin, 117*(3), 387–403.

Chapter 9
Can't Live with You, Can't Live Without You: How to Tailor Coaching for Dyads with Ambivalent/Resistant Attachment

This chapter discusses the challenges of working with ambivalent/resistant parent–child dyads. I describe how to recognize ambivalent/resistant attachment, factors associated with the development of ambivalent/resistant attachment, and how this pattern of attachment may be adaptive for the child. I describe how to tailor IoWA-PCIT to address the emotional and behavioral problems of children in ambivalent/resistant dyads and the course of treatment with ambivalent/resistant dyads.

As noted earlier in this book, each child's path to developing a strategy for getting their attachment needs met by their parent is unique. However, research on common paths to developing an ambivalent/resistant pattern of attachment can help us develop hypotheses about how this pattern of attachment may have developed in any particular dyad we're coaching and why this strategy may be adaptive for the child.

How to Recognize Ambivalent/Resistant Pattern of Attachment

In ambivalent/resistant dyads, the child is preoccupied with their parent (Ainsworth et al., 1978; Beebe et al., 2010; Beebe & Lachmann, 2014; Cassidy & Marvin, 1992; Main, 2000). This has been described as hyperactivation of the attachment system (Main, 2000). In other words, it is as though the attachment system is set on high alert, always ready to be activated. Every stressor, for example, entering a new room, a stranger entering, and the parent indicating they are going to leave, is a signal to activate the attachment system. If one were to only look at the attachment side of the attachment–exploration balance, one might describe the child as "too attached." The child is often close to the parent and may appear clingy and reluctant to be away from the parent. However, while the child and parent are physically close, their relationship appears tense. The child is often whiny or angry and there is an undercurrent of conflict in their interaction. This pattern is most striking during reunions with the parent. Despite the child's significant distress at being separated from the parent, the child continues to remain distressed when the parent returns. Some infants and young children may even act angry when their parent returns—sometimes even hitting the parent when they return. One of the most striking aspects of ambivalent/resistant dyads is the child's rejection of the parent's efforts to calm the child through hugs or other positive physical touch. Children will continue to exhibit distress and squirm or push away as their parent attempts to hug them.

There are two types of ambivalent/resistant attachment that are distinguished primarily by whether the resistance is active or passive. In ambivalent/resistant attachment relationships where the resistance is active, the parent–child struggle is prominent. The child is extremely distressed during the separation but actively resists the parent's attempts to interact with them when the parent returns. The child frequently appears angry and frustrated in interactions with the parent and unresponsive to the parent's attempts to engage them.

In ambivalent/resistant attachment relationships where the resistance is passive, both exploratory behavior and attempts to engage the parent are limited. For example, the infant may cry but not make efforts to move toward the parent. In preschool-aged children, the passive resistance is exhibited through immature behavior such as baby talk, clinging to the parent, or wanting to be held. The child is preoccupied with the parent but does not seem to enjoy interactions with the parent or feel soothed by the parent's presence.

Development of Ambivalent/Resistant Attachment Pattern

Research on the development of the ambivalent/resistant pattern of attachment suggests several early factors in the parent's response to the child's attachment signals that may contribute to the development of this pattern. Parents of infants and young children with ambivalent/resistant attachment patterns are more inconsistent in their response to their child's attachment needs than parents in secure dyads (Ainsworth et al., 1978; Main, 2000). They can be sensitively responsive to their child's attachment needs at times and fail to respond sensitively at other times. Parents who are stressed and report more anxiety about being separated from their child are also more likely to have an ambivalent/resistant attachment relationship with their child (Scher & Mayseless, 2000). Factors associated with the parent's stress level may also contribute to an ambivalent/resistant relationship with their child. For example, parents who work longer hours are more likely to have an ambivalent/resistant attachment relationship (Scher & Mayseless, 2000). Placement in a group childcare setting has also been associated with this pattern of attachment (Scher & Mayseless, 2000).

Clinically, I have also seen ambivalent/resistant attachment in children who experience frequent moves between parents. Frequent moves between parents can occur in joint custody situations, in childcare settings where there is frequent turnover in providers, and when children in foster care have frequent moves between placements. This reminds me that an important part of sensitively responsive care is the parent being able to read and understand the child's cues—a job that is made more difficult without the consistency of a daily routine with the child.

The research I have found the most helpful in understanding the development of this pattern is the microanalytic analyses of interactions between 4-month-old infants and their mothers conducted by Beatrice Beebe and Frank Lachmann (Beebe et al., 2010, 2016; Beebe & Lachmann, 2014). During face-to-face interactions with their 4-month-old infant, mothers in future ambivalent/resistant dyads engage in a type of interaction that Beebe and Lachmann (2014) describe as "chase and dodge."

An understanding of the chase and dodge dynamic begins with an understanding of how babies use gaze aversion. Infants look away from their parent's face as a way to self-regulate when they become overstimulated by the very hard work of focusing their attention on interacting with their parent. However, in dyads that will become ambivalent/resistant, the parent will "chase" the baby by vocalizing, touching the baby, and trying to make eye contact when the baby attempts to look away. The baby will respond by trying to "dodge" the parent's attempts to engage by trying to look away from the parent (Beebe et al., 2010, 2016; Beebe & Lachmann, 2014). During my workshops, I often have therapists role-play the chase and dodge dynamic. When pretending to be a baby whose parent will not let them look away, their visceral response is an indication of how anxiety-provoking it is to feel trapped in this dynamic. When pretending to be a parent who is "chasing" the baby's gaze, therapists have a recognition of how hard the parents in ambivalent/resistant dyads are trying and how frustrating it is when they feel as though their efforts are not rewarded.

The research conducted by Beatrice Beebe and her colleagues also helped me make sense of a phenomenon I found puzzling—the tendency of infants and young children in ambivalent/resistant relationships to resist their parent's affectionate interactions. During face-to-face interactions with their 4-month-old infant, mothers in future ambivalent/resistant dyads became progressively less positive, more active, and more intrusive in their interactions with their infant (e.g., scratching, pulling, pushing, and poking the infant) (Beebe et al., 2010). The mother's touch seemed to be focused on getting the baby to pay attention to her rather than a response to the child's distress and need for soothing, a distinct contrast to maternal touch in secure dyads. Consequently, by 4 months of age, infants who were later classified as ambivalent/resistant had already begun to "tune out" their mother's touch—whether that touch was positive or negative (Beebe & Lachmann, 2014). These future ambivalent/resistant infants are less likely to protest when their mother's touch becomes intrusive and less likely to express positive emotions when their mother's touch becomes more affectionate. They have learned at an early age not to trust their parent's touch.

The infants who would later be classified as ambivalent/resistant were also overly vigilant to their mother's face during face-to-face interactions (Beebe & Lachmann, 2014). By 4 months of age, the baby has already learned to watch their mother carefully for clues as to how to get their attachment needs met and clues that their mother is becoming intrusive. This need to be vigilant to the parent's face leaves less time for visually exploring the environment—the precursor to exploring the environment in other ways.

How Ambivalent/Resistant Attachment May Be Adaptive for the Child

For children in an ambivalent/resistant attachment relationship, intense focus on the relationship is their way of getting their attachment needs met. The child is acutely focused on the parent in order to get their attachment needs met in the face of a mixture of responsive and unresponsive parenting or frequent moves between caregivers. This strategy ensures the child doesn't miss out on any opportunities to connect with a parent. This intense focus on the parent is also protective—it means the child is prepared for the parent becoming too intrusive.

Prevalence of Ambivalent/Resistant Attachment Pattern

Approximately 10% of child–parent dyads in community samples exhibit an ambivalent/resistant attachment (Booth-LaForce & Roisman, 2014; Kochanska & Kim, 2013; Moss et al., 2004; van Ijzendoorn et al., 1999). Approximately 20% of child–parent dyads referred to me for IoWA-PCIT exhibit an ambivalent/resistant attachment.

How to Promote Secure Attachment in Ambivalent/Resistant Dyads

In order for the child to be able to become less preoccupied with the relationship with the parent and engage in more exploration, the child needs for their parent to provide more support for exploration. That is, the parent needs to provide a secure base. The child needs to know the parent supports their exploration. The parent also needs to be available as a safe haven when the child meets challenges and becomes distressed when venturing out.

As with coaching secure dyads, Child-Directed Interaction (CDI) coaching (described in Chap. 4) can focus on the parent providing prompt, consistent, and appropriate responses to the child's attachment signals. In ambivalent/resistant dyads, it is especially important to be attentive to the child's need to have their exploration supported. Parents can do this in CDI by describing what the child is doing. Behavior descriptions are a way for the parent to communicate to the child that they are available so the child can feel more comfortable exploring.

Another focus of CDI is reducing the parent's frequency of intrusive and negative touch. More than in other dyads, I find parents in ambivalent/resistant dyads engage in intrusive physical interactions such as leaning into their child's space and negative touch such as tugging on their child's arm. Not surprisingly, children in ambivalent/resistant dyads seem less responsive to positive physical touch such as when the parent wants to give them a hug or get them to sit on their lap. In order for the child to be able to "take in" the parent's positive touch and soothing, the parent needs to reduce the use of intrusive and negative touch.

I try to decrease a parent's intrusive interactions by focusing on the positive opposite—pointing out when they are giving their child space. I say things like "Great job of sitting back and letting him solve that on his own. I know how hard it is for you to see him struggle."

My coaching is more directive in situations where the parent is engaging in negative touch. Like criticism, I consider negative touch to be especially damaging to the parent–child relationship and prioritize this type of interaction as one where I want to be more directive. If the negative touch occurs in a situation that does not involve a behavior problem, for example, the parent wants the child to play with them, I'll provide reassurance and coach the parent to follow the child's lead. For example, "It's okay if he doesn't want to play with the toy you're playing with. He is learning to be more independent which is such an important skill at his age. Keep describing what he is doing. Your support is so important to him while he is learning to play on his own."

If the negative touch occurs when the parent is trying to correct a minor problem such as the child playing roughly with the toys, I will remind the parent they can use an active ignore instead of physically intervening in their child's behavior. For example, "I see you're concerned about how roughly he is playing with the toys. I appreciate you wanting him to be gentler with my toys, but I think this is the type of situation where you can use an active ignore. Go ahead and pick up a couple of toys and describe your own play. Say I'm having the horse and the giraffe take a walk together." If the negative touch occurs when the parent is trying to correct the behavior that is dangerous or destructive, I will remind the parent of the rules for managing dangerous or destructive behavior during CDI. For example, "I see you're concerned about him trying to climb on the table. Remind him that climbing on the table is dangerous and if he climbs on the table special play will be over."

Another way of promoting secure attachment in CDI is by encouraging the parent to wait until the child asks for help or invites physical affection. In this way, the parent learns to act as a safe haven in response to the child's cues, not in response to the parent's needs.

Parent-Directed Interaction (PDI) (described in Chap. 5) is especially important in helping ambivalent/resistant dyads move to a more secure relationship. The experience of having the parent communicate clear expectations and set appropriate limits leads to a more rewarding relationship for both the parent and child. PDI is an important step in addressing the aggression toward the parent that is often a feature of ambivalent/resistant attachment relationships. PDI is also especially challenging for ambivalent/resistant dyads. It is important to move slowly in rolling out PDI for ambivalent/resistant dyads, recognizing the anxiety this stage of treatment can evoke for both the parent and child.

Course of IoWA-PCIT with Ambivalent/Resistant Dyads

In my experience, dyads with an ambivalent/resistant pattern of attachment make significant progress in IoWA-PCIT, moving from clinically significant disruptive behavior and anxiety to age-typical emotional and behavioral regulation. Most importantly, aggression toward the parent, a prominent characteristic of these dyads, is eliminated at the end of treatment. One of the reasons for this success is that, in my experience, ambivalent/resistant dyads do not drop out of treatment—they hang in there until the problematic interactions have been addressed. Although this is an accurate description of the outcomes in ambivalent/resistant dyads, it does not capture the process of working with these dyads. Working with ambivalent/resistant dyads can be challenging. In the middle of treatment with an ambivalent/resistant dyad, it is easy to become discouraged.

Children in ambivalent/resistant dyads will repeatedly return to their "go to" behaviors of whining and being easily frustrated. These behaviors have worked in the past to get their attachment needs met, and they are reluctant to give them up. Ignoring these behaviors will lead to escalation of emotions and behavior until they learn more reliable ways of getting their attachment needs met. Under stress, when their attachment needs are heightened, they will often return to these behaviors. Because of this, helping these dyads learn a new pattern of getting their attachment needs met often feels like two steps forward and one step back.

Positive physical touch is often confusing and dysregulating for young children in ambivalent/resistant relationships at the beginning of treatment. As coaching focuses on parents becoming less intrusive with their physical touch, we see children begin to seek out more physical affection from their parent and the affection becomes more regulating.

One of the most rewarding moments in coaching ambivalent/resistant dyads is the emergence of effective soothing and co-regulation. As children in ambivalent/resistant dyads begin to have more opportunities to demonstrate their competence in exploration, they also have moments where they seek out assistance from their parent when frustrated or upset. When the child seeks a brief hug and then returns to play, I know they're beginning to move toward a more secure and rewarding pattern of interaction with their parent.

In my clinical experience, it takes longer for ambivalent/resistant dyads to make significant changes in their interactions than secure dyads. It is not unusual for ambivalent/resistant dyads to spend more than 20 sessions in IoWA-PCIT, and the majority spend more than 30 sessions.

Countertransference/Common Pitfalls

There is a quality of "Don't you dare give me what I'm asking for" in ambivalent/resistant dyads that is frustrating to observe. When we lose sight of the inconsistency that likely contributed to the development of this pattern of attachment, we can easily become frustrated with a child who seems to be chronically upset and unresponsive to their parent's efforts.

When working with the ambivalent immature subtype of this pattern of attachment, it is easy to fall into a sense of helplessness. Even Mary Ainsworth and her colleagues (Ainsworth et al., 1978) sound a bit helpless and critical in the description of ambivalent immature dyads. When describing this pattern in infants, they note: "Passivity is notoriously resistant to treatment and reversal in later years. The passive-aggressive personality—the criteria for which fit our C_2 babies very well, even in the first year of life—is obviously associated with profound problems in dealing with the issues and challenges of later life. From our point of view the passivity of the C_2 infant seems to be deeply rooted. An infant whose mother almost never responds contingently to his signals must have a profound lack of confidence in his ability to have any effective control of what happens to him" (Ainsworth et al., 1978). It is important to recognize the sense of helplessness engendered in us when working with these dyads—a taste of the child's experience of the world.

The Bottom Line

IoWA-PCIT is highly effective in reducing disruptive behavior in ambivalent/resistant dyads. A primary goal when working with ambivalent/resistant dyads is to help the dyad become more comfortable with the child exploring the environment. The positive parent verbalizations that are a feature of CDI are an important way for the parent to communicate support for exploration. PDI is especially important for dyads with ambivalent/resistant attachment. However, PDI tends to take longer with ambivalent/resistant dyads than it does with more secure dyads. When working with ambivalent/resistant dyads, it is important to be patient and keep space for the possibility there will be some regressions along with overall growth.

References

Ainsworth, M., Blehar, M., Waters, E., & Wall, S. (1978). *Patterns of attachment: A psychological study of the strange situation*. Erlbaum.

Beebe, B., Cohen, P., & Lachmann, F. (2016). *The mother-infant interaction picture book*. Norton.

Beebe, B., Jaffe, J., Markese, S., Buck, K., Chen, H., Cohen, P., ... Feldstein, S. (2010). The origins of 12-month attachment: A microanalysis of 4-month mother-infant interaction. *Attachment & Human Development, 12*(1–2), 3–141.

Beebe, B., & Lachmann, F. (2014). *The origins of attachment: Infant research and adult treatment.* Routledge.

Booth-LaForce, C., & Roisman, G. (2014). The adult attachment interview: Psychometrics, stability and change from infancy and developmental origins. *Monographs of the Society for Research in Child Development, 79*(3), 1–185.

Cassidy, J., & Marvin, R. (1992). *Attachment organization in preschool children: Procedures and coding manual.* University of Virginia.

Kochanska, G., & Kim, S. (2013). Early attachment organization with both parents and future behavior problems: From infancy to middle childhood. *Child Development, 84*(1), 283–296.

Main, M. (2000). The organized categories of infant, child, and adult attachment: Flexible vs. inflexible attention under attachment-related stress. *Journal of the American Psychoanalytic Association, 48*, 1055–1096.

Moss, E., Cyr, C., & Dubois-Comtois, K. (2004). Attachment at early school age and developmental risk: Examining family contexts and behavior problems of controlling-caregiving, controlling-punitive, and behaviorally disorganized children. *Developmental Psychology, 40*(4), 519–532.

Scher, A., & Mayseless, O. (2000). Mothers of anxious/ambivalent infants: Maternal characteristics and child-care context. *Child Development, 71*, 1629–1639.

van Ijzendoorn, M., Schungel, C., & Bakermans-Kranenburg, M. J. (1999). Disorganized attachment in early childhood: Meta-analysis of precursors, concomitants, and sequelae. *Development and Psychopathology, 11*, 225–249.

Chapter 10
Mired in Relationships: How to Tailor Coaching for Parents with Preoccupied Attachment

This chapter discusses how to adapt parent coaching for parents who have a preoccupied working model of attachment. Particular attention is paid to recognizing how the parent's preoccupied attachment colors perceptions of the child and the therapist and how to take this into account when coaching parents with preoccupied attachment.

How to Recognize Preoccupied Working Model of Attachment in Parents

As noted in the previous chapter, infants and young children in ambivalent/resistant dyads appear preoccupied with their parents. Thus, it makes sense that the type of internal working model of attachment seen most frequently in the parents of these dyads is labeled preoccupied (George et al., 1984; Main, 2000). In the Adult Attachment Interview (AAI), this preoccupation presents as excessively long conversation turns when discussing attachment-related experiences (George et al., 1984; Main, 2000). Adults with a preoccupied working model of attachment are preoccupied with early attachment experiences, vacillating between positive and negative evaluations of their parents. There are three subtypes of preoccupied attachment: passive, angry/conflicted, and fearfully preoccupied with traumatic events.

Research on how individuals with preoccupied attachment communicate with their therapists indicates this preoccupation is also exhibited in communications with therapists (Talia et al., 2014, 2015). Somewhat surprisingly, preoccupied patients tend to engage in fewer proximity-seeking communications with their therapists than more secure patients (Talia et al., 2014, 2015). In other words, although preoccupied patients seem to want support from their therapist, they are less likely to directly ask for help or advice from their therapist or even to directly disclose distress. In addition, they resist their therapist's help. Some of the ways they directly resist their therapist's interventions are by changing to another distressing topic when the therapist tries to explore their distress or continuing to focus on their distress without acknowledging the therapist's intervention (Talia et al., 2014, 2015). Preoccupied patients also tend to enlist the therapist's agreement with their opinion or quote someone else as a way of reinforcing their opinion (Talia et al., 2014, 2015). Just as children in ambivalent/resistant relationships have difficulty with exploration, preoccupied patients have difficulty exploring new ideas or opinions, seeking instead to enlist support for their current ideas. Preoccupied patients also tend to change topics abruptly, rapidly change their views of a problem or situation, and speak in vague generalities (Talia et al., 2014, 2015). In other words, their conversation can be difficult to follow.

Research on how preoccupied mothers respond to their infants indicates they tend to become more intrusive when their baby is calm but to withdraw when their baby is distressed (Haltigan et al., 2014). This pattern of responding keeps the child focused on the parent and keeps distress as the focus of the relationship.

How Preoccupied Working Model May Be Adaptive

Like ambivalent/resistant attachment, preoccupied attachment is a strategy of hyperactivation of the attachment system (Main, 2000). That is, it is a way of being in relationship where there is an intense focus on the attachment relationship. Preoccupied attachment may be adaptive for the parent as it allows them to get their attachment needs met by staying focused on attachment relationships.

Prevalence of Preoccupied Attachment

In community samples, 3–10% of adults have a preoccupied working model of attachment (Bakermans-Kranenburg & van Ijzendoorn, 2009; Booth-LaForce & Roisman, 2014; Caspers et al., 2007). Rates are somewhat higher (15–30%) in psychotherapy patients (Levy et al., 2006; Talia et al., 2015).

Course of IoWA-PCIT with Preoccupied Parents

When coaching parents with a preoccupied working model of attachment, it is important to remember their tendency to present as vulnerable and incompetent in order to get their attachment needs met. Preoccupied parents struggle with their child exploring due to feelings of rejection and not being needed by the child when the child is not focused on interacting with them.

The majority of parents with a preoccupied working model of attachment describe feeling abandoned and ignored by their own parents, a pattern they do not want to repeat with their child. Although parents with a preoccupied working model of attachment describe feeling ignored by their own parents when they were children, their parents are often very much involved in their lives as adults—and in the lives of their children. Despite, or perhaps because of, this ongoing involvement in their lives, preoccupied parents typically continue to feel a lack of support from their parents. To me, this illustrates how the parent's ongoing sense of not having their needs met is characterized by a lack of emotional support and validation rather than other types of support.

Due to the hyperactivation of the attachment system seen in individuals with preoccupied attachment, working with these parents can be emotionally exhausting. I think of it as the parent spreading their negative affect around and infecting others with their negative emotionality. I experienced this myself when writing this chapter. I began to feel like a fraud—thinking to myself, who am I to be writing a chapter on working with parents with preoccupied attachment? I'm not sure I have been helpful to parents with preoccupied attachment. As I wrote, I thought of all the ways these parents had reminded me that I hadn't been helpful enough to them and their child. So, I decided to look at my data. I analyzed the outcomes for all the ambivalent/resistant dyads where I thought the parent had a preoccupied working model of attachment. I was stunned. I found that for these dyads there had been significant declines in disruptive behavior as assessed by parent ratings on the Eyberg Child Behavior Inventory (ECBI) (Eyberg & Pincus, 1999). In fact, the amount of improvement was actually somewhat greater than for dyads that were securely attached. Although the researcher in me hastens to add this is probably not a statistically significant difference, it did make me realize how the experience of working with these dyads is different than the outcomes. I should also note that, in my experience, these parents tend to spend more time in IoWA-PCIT than those parents with more secure working models of attachment. Again, while the length of time parents with preoccupied attachment spend in therapy can feel discouraging, I have come to believe that it is important to take the time that it takes for the parent to experience a new way of being in relationship.

One of the most important tasks when working with parents with preoccupied attachment is supporting them through moments when their child is exploring. It is important for them to have our support when their child is exploring the environment so they can begin to see that their child needs them for exploration as well as for attachment.

Just as the parent is learning that the child needs them during exploration and moments of displaying their competence, parents with preoccupied attachment need our support when they are competently handling a situation with their child and enjoying time with their child. They need to learn that we have their back when they are doing well—not just when they are focusing on problems. It can be difficult for parents with preoccupied attachment to acknowledge their gains in competence and their child's improvement during IoWA-PCIT as this also involves acknowledging the role they had in their child's difficulties (Biermann, 2021). They tend to perceive these changes through a negative lens—that is, if their child does better when they respond differently, then maybe the problems were their fault.

When coaching parents with preoccupied attachment, we need to strike a balance between validating concerns and recognizing strengths. Below is an example of how a therapist might address the tendency of a parent with a preoccupied working model of attachment to focus on negative affect and problems in her relationship with her child. In this example, during the check-in at the beginning of the session, the parent describes an incident the night before where her child had an extended tantrum over what she had made for supper. The tantrum escalated to the point where she and her child were yelling at each other. The therapist listens attentively during the check-in but does not ask questions or offer advice on how to handle future tantrums. She keeps the check-in brief, has the parent put the communication device in her ear, and leaves the room so the child and parent can begin CDI. During the 5 minutes of CDI coding, there are warm interactions between the child and parent and the parent exhibits a high level of CDI skills. The following exchange occurs at the end of the 5 minutes of coding.

Therapist to parent: "Tell Patrick you will be listening to me for a minute."
Parent to child: "I'm going to listen to the therapist for a minute."
Child to parent: "OK. Can I listen to the therapist?"
Parent hands the communication device to child.
Therapist to child: "You're doing a really nice job of playing with your mom this morning.
Child beams, giggles, and hands the communication device back to parent."
Analysis: Whether to address the child directly over the communication device is a clinical decision. The therapist made a clinical decision to speak directly with the child for the following reasons: (1) Although the session had started with the parent complaining to the therapist about the child's behavior in front of the child, the child had regrouped and played positively with the parent, so the therapist wanted to provide additional reinforcement to the child. (2) Since the parent had handed the communication device to the child, it would be difficult for the therapist to not respond.
Therapist to parent: "You did an excellent job with your CDI skills today—fifteen reflections, eight behavior descriptions, and eight labeled praises. I am so impressed with your ability to come in and do such great CDI after what happened last night."
Analysis: The therapist leads with a focus on the parent's competence while also acknowledging the negative affect and complaining—the parent's usual way of connecting with attachment figures.
Therapist to parent: "I noticed that Patrick told you he was having a bit of difficulty with getting the train track together. Let's look for opportunities to praise him for using his words to let you know when he's struggling. When you get into a situation like last night, it may be beyond words, even for you. But we can begin to work on him using his words in stressful situations."

Analysis: The therapist again acknowledges the difficulties of the previous evening. She presents an idea for how to begin addressing this during coaching while acknowledging the difficulties of using words during stressful situations.
Child to parent: "Can we play again?"
Therapist to parent: "I'm done. You can go back to playing with him. I was rambling a bit." *Analysis: Acknowledges that she may have spent too much time with explanations instead of coaching.*
Child to parent: "I'll take this part of the train and you can have this part."
Therapist to parent: "He is getting so good at sharing."
Analysis: The therapist makes an observation about child's positive behavior and positive changes in child.
Parent to child: "Thank you for sharing with me."
Therapist to parent: "Great labeled praise!"
Child happily pushes his train around the track while singing and smiling at his mother.
Therapist to parent: "Kids have such short memories. It's clear how difficult your evening was and now he's singing and happy."
Analysis: The therapist again acknowledges the two sides of their relationship. She acknowledges how difficult the previous evening was when the child and parent were both struggling with their emotional regulation. However, she also acknowledges that there is more to their relationship than the struggle—there are also these moments of joy and shared positive affect.

Countertransference/Common Pitfalls

In addition to discussing what to do when working with parents with preoccupied attachment, I also want to give you a sense of what not to do. Or, more realistically, how to avoid getting into the same pitfalls repeatedly with a parent. In our attempts to meet the attachment needs of parents with a preoccupied working model of attachment, there can be a tendency to focus too much on the parent's concerns and negative affect regarding their child. I still find myself falling into these pitfalls but over time have learned to spend less time repeating them.

When working with parents with preoccupied working models of attachment, I often feel pressure to rescue the parent by solving the problem for them or by switching therapeutic approaches. These are the parents where I find myself spending a significant amount of time discussing the parent's concerns about their child, friends, or other family members. This is part of the countertransference pull that I need to acknowledge to myself but not become mired in. It is easy to imagine how the exchange above could have gone differently if I had focused on the parent's negative affect and concerns rather than moving to CDI coaching. As I focused on dissecting and rehashing the difficult events of the evening, the parent would likely have continued to focus on the negative affect. As the parent continued to focus on her negative affect, it is likely she would have become more distressed and upset (what we call hyperactivation of attachment). Her child would have responded to hearing about his negative behavior by becoming more upset in order to get his attachment needs met. Instead, I was able to give the parent a new experience, getting support for her competence. This allowed her to focus on an aspect of her child she tended not to notice—his resilience and positive affect.

PDI is especially challenging for parents with preoccupied working model of attachment. They do not like to be in a position of authority and would prefer that their child do things without being told to do them. Below is an example of how a therapist might coach a parent with preoccupied working model of attachment during the PDI phase of treatment. In this example, the session began with the parent complaining to the therapist about the child's failure to pick up his toys at home. The parent described an incident that occurred the evening before when the child's failure to pick up toys escalated into the child throwing toys. The exchange below occurred about 15 minutes into the session, after the therapist had coded CDI for 5 minutes and coached CDI for 5 minutes. Given the difficulties described by the parent, the therapist decided not to code PDI and to focus on coaching PDI instead.

Therapist to parent: "What do you think about challenging him by giving him a clean-up command?"
Analysis: The therapist gives the parent agency to decide whether she wants to work on the problem she described at the beginning of the session. She communicates that she understands cleanup commands are challenging for the parent and her child.
Parent to child: "Please put these blocks in the box."
Therapist to parent: "Nice direct command."
Analysis: The therapist praises parent for giving an authoritative, effective command. The therapist notes to herself that this is a big command for a child who had difficulty with picking up toys at home but decides to wait to comment on this.
Child to parent: (While picking up blocks and putting them in the box.) "This is so boring."
Therapist to parent: "Nice job of ignoring the verbiage. I agree with him. Picking up toys is boring."
Analysis: The therapist praises parent for not getting into an argument with the child. She communicates to the parent that it is possible to both empathize with your child's feelings and set appropriate boundaries.
Therapist to parent: "He did it! Yay!"
Analysis: The therapist expresses enthusiasm for child's achievement.
Parent to child: "Thank you for picking up the blocks! Now we have more room to play with the trains."
Therapist to parent: "Great labeled praise for compliance. And, you added a reason for why he needed to pick up the blocks! I am so impressed you were willing to practice this today."
Analysis: The therapist praises parent's competence.
Child to parent: "Let's play with the trains!" (Gives parent a quick hug and begins pushing a train around the track.)

Therapist to parent: "Ahhhh. It's nice to see how proud he is of himself when he is able to follow your command. Go back to CDI and I'll have you give another command in a couple of minutes."
Analysis: The therapist describes child's positive reaction to being competent at picking up toys.

Admittedly, it is tough to shift from talking through issues with parents with preoccupied attachment to coaching them through the issues. If it seems the parent is continually pushing for more time to talk with you at the beginning of the session, you may want to consider scheduling a parent-only session (without the child present) to provide more support for the parent. However, even in these sessions, it is important the focus be on giving the parent the type of support they need—that is, supporting the expansion of their strategies for getting their attachment needs met. In other words, it is important to balance support for their concerns with support for their competence. Reviewing video clips where the parent has been competent in managing their child's behavior problems can be useful in reinforcing this expansion of their skills.

Some of the ways the parent's preoccupied working model can make it difficult to provide support are the ways in which they resist help. For example, parents with a preoccupied working model of attachment often express dissatisfaction with treatment. When the therapist expresses empathy about their concerns, they often change topics and bring up something else they are distressed about—often another person in their life—rather than discussing their concerns about treatment. Another way in which parents with preoccupied attachment resist the help they crave is by bringing in the opinions of other people about the treatment approach—their parents, their child's teacher, their minister— everyone seems to have an opinion about the problems with the treatment approach.

I'll be honest—more than once I have found myself arguing with someone who is not in the room. In case you're not sure what I mean by arguing with someone who is not in the room, first, congratulations for avoiding this particular misstep. This is where I find myself explaining to the grandparent, minister, or someone else I've never met why I disagree with them—for example, "I think your minister is wrong about the need to spank your child more." Or, "Have you explained to your son's teacher that it may take a while before his behavior at school improves?" I have learned to recognize when I'm about to start arguing with someone who is not in the room, to step back, and to try to help the parent voice her own concerns. For example, I say things like "I wonder what your thoughts are about spanking." Or, "I wonder what it is like to have your mother criticize your approach to parenting," or simply, "It sounds like it has been a really tough week. I'm sorry you had to deal with him having such an extreme tantrum at your in-law's."

Basically, I try to communicate that conflict and disagreement is something we can discuss—not just a strategy for being in relationship. Also, by trying to help the parent find their voice with me, I hope to help them find their voice in discussions with others. Once they are able to own the concerns about the treatment approach, they can begin to own the successes as well. As they begin to see the positive impact of CDI and PDI on their interactions with their child, they begin to have greater trust in their ability to know what is best for their child.

A psychoanalytic concept I find useful in understanding the experience of working with preoccupied parents is projective identification (Ogden, 1982), a concept introduced by Melanie Klein (Klein, 1946, 1955) (one of John Bowlby's mentors). Early attachment trauma, especially attachment trauma that occurs when children are preverbal, can literally not be talked about—people do not have words for it. So, they communicate what happened through enactments—acting out the pattern of attachment trauma with others. As part of communicating what they experienced to someone else, they put the feeling they had to deal with into the other person. This whole concept has a bit of a mystical quality to it—especially for those of us who like to communicate in words and numbers. I believe it is a real phenomenon and we are just beginning to understand the specifics of how this nonverbal communication works.

What I know is that the feelings engendered in us when working with these families are real. And when we pay attention to those feelings and accept them, we are able to do better work with these parents. When consulting on cases where the parent has a preoccupied working model of attachment, I have noticed the way in which the affective temperature of the consultation group rises when discussing these families. It's as though we begin to communicate for the members of the family, trying to get our own needs to be acknowledged and heard in the group in the way the family does.

It can be tricky to discuss the experience of projective identification and parallel process that can arise in consultation groups. This discussion starts by acknowledging the different experiences we bring to our work and to the group. None of us want to feel we have been caught up in someone else's drama or that there are aspects of this drama that may relate to our own attachment histories. And, of course, it doesn't feel like someone else's drama, it feels like our drama. It actually becomes our drama until we can talk about the experience, reflect on it, and realize we can choose different ways of communicating with each other in the group. I used to think about these types of group discussions as a distraction from our work with families. I now realize this is one of the most important aspects of our work with families. Becoming caught up in a family drama and working through it with our colleagues can help us see new pathways forward.

So far, I have been discussing how to coach a preoccupied parent who has an ambivalent/resistant attachment relationship with their child. Due to the strong association between the parent and child's working model, this is the most common combination. On a few occasions, I have worked with preoccupied parents where the child's working model didn't "match" the parent's preoccupation with relationships. I want to touch briefly on the experience of coaching these less common combinations.

Preoccupied Parent in a Secure Relationship with Their Child

I have had the opportunity to work with some dyads where the child has a secure attachment with the parent although the parent appears to have a preoccupied working model of attachment. In these dyads, the child is appropriately assertive in communicating their needs for attachment and their needs for exploration, despite the parent's preoccupation with their relationship with the child, me, and others in their life. When coaching preoccupied parents in a secure relationship with their child, I am able to help the parent see that self-assertiveness and competence are healthy and to celebrate the ways in which they have facilitated their child's exploration and attachment.

Preoccupied Parent in an Avoidant Relationship with Their Child

Some children, when faced with an inconsistently responsive parent, develop a strategy of self-reliance and independence rather than the clinginess and aggression we typically see in dyads where the parent has a preoccupied pattern of attachment. These can be challenging dyads to work with because the parent is so focused on their own attachment needs and the child is so focused on exploration, it is difficult to find the middle ground. Helping the parent and child meet in the middle is exactly what we need to do with these dyads. For these dyads, it is especially important to note any ways in which the child communicates their need for help to the parent and prompt the parent to respond to the child's need. These cues can be especially subtle in these dyads. For example, if a child is struggling with a toy with their back to the parent, turns and holds it out to the parent, you might say, "It looks like he wants your help with that toy. Tell him you can help him with that toy."

In these dyads, it is especially important that the parent recognizes the child still needs them when they are exploring. You might make observations like "He just looked at you before he put the train on the track. He wants to know you approve of what he is doing. When you describe what he is doing that lets him know you approve."

The Bottom Line

When working with parents with preoccupied attachment, our goal is to teach them a different way of communicating their attachment needs and a different way of being in relationship—both in their relationship with us and their relationship with their child. That is, we want them to learn that supporting their child's exploration is as important as exploring their child's attachment. We also want them to learn to embrace their own competence and capacity for self-regulation. The challenging aspect of coaching parents with preoccupied attachment is the extent to which they are stuck in a particular view of themselves and relationships—one where they must struggle in order to remain in relationship. What we have on our side when working with preoccupied parents is their strong interest in relationships and their commitment to building a more positive relationship with their child.

References

Bakermans-Kranenburg, M., & van Ijzendoorn, M. (2009). The first 10,000 adult attachment interviews: Distributions of adult attachment representations in clinical and non-clinical groups. *Attachment & Human Development, 11*(3), 223–263.

Biermann, A. (2021, May). personal communication.

Booth-LaForce, C., & Roisman, G. (2014). The adult attachment interview: Psychometrics, stability and change from infancy and developmental origins. *Monographs of the Society for Research in Child Development, 79*(3), 1–185.

Caspers, K. M., Yucuis, R., Troutman, B., Arndt, S., & Langbehn, D. (2007). A sibling adoption study of adult attachment: The influence of shared environment on attachment state of mind. *Attachment & Human Development, 9*(4), 375–391.

Eyberg, S., & Pincus, D. (1999). *Eyberg child behavior inventory and Sutter-Eyberg student behavior inventory – revised.* Psychological Assessment Resources.

George, C., Kaplan, N., & Main, M. (1984). *Adult attachment interview.* University of California.

Haltigan, J., Leerkes, E., Supple, A., & Calkins, S. (2014). Infant negative affect and maternal interactive behavior during the still-face procedure: The moderating role of adult attachment states of mind. *Attachment & Human Development, 16*(2), 149–173.

Klein, M. (1946). Notes on some schizoid mechanisms. In *Envy and gratitude and other works, 1946–1963* (pp. 1–24). Delacorte Press.

Klein, M. (1955). On identification. In *Envy and gratitude and other works, 1946–1963* (pp. 141–175). Delacorte Press.

Levy, K., Meehan, K., Kelly, K., Reynoson, J., Weber, M., Clarkin, J., & Kernberg, O. (2006). Change in attachment patterns and reflective function in a randomized control trial of transference-focused pyschotherapy for borderline personality disorder. *Journal of Consulting and Clinical Psychology, 74*(6), 1027–1040.

Main, M. (2000). The organized categories of infant, child, and adult attachment: Flexible vs. inflexible attention under attachment-related stress. *Journal of the American Psychoanalytic Association, 48,* 1055–1096.

Ogden, T. (1982). *Projective Identification & Psychotherapeutic Technique.* Jason Aronson Inc.

Talia, A., Daniel, S., Miller-Bottome, M., Brambilla, D., Miccoli, D., Safran, J., & Lingiardi, V. (2014). AAI predicts patients' in-session interpersonal behavior and discourse: A "move to the level of the relation" for attachment-informed psychotherapy research. *Attachment & Human Development, 16*(2), 192–209.

Talia, A., Miller-Bottome, M., & Daniel, S. (2015). Assessing attachment in psychotherapy: Validation study of the patient attachment coding system. *Clinical Psychology & Psychotherapy, 24,* 149–161.

Chapter 11
Going It Alone: How to Tailor Coaching for Dyads with Avoidant Attachment

This chapter discusses the challenges of working with avoidant parent–child dyads. Factors associated with this pattern of attachment, how it may be adaptive for the child, and how to address the emotional and behavioral problems of children in avoidant dyads are described.

How to Recognize Avoidant Pattern of Attachment

In avoidant infant–parent dyads, the infant may physically turn away from the parent, busying themselves with a toy, when the parent enters the room after a brief absence (Ainsworth et al., 1978; Main, 2000). In regard to the attachment–exploration balance, the balance in avoidant dyads involves too much focus on independence and not enough focus on attachment. This is referred to as deactivation of the attachment system (Main, 2000). In other words, the child turns off their needs for comfort and support when distressed in order to maintain their relationship with the parent. If one were to only look at the attachment side of the attachment–exploration balance, one might describe the child as "not attached." In fact, the avoidant attachment pattern is a strategy for maintaining a relationship with the parent—the strategy of not being too needy in order to maintain proximity to the parent. If one were to only look at the exploration side of the attachment–exploration balance, one might describe the child as "competent" and "independent," characteristics that are much admired in many families and cultures.

By the time the child is in preschool, there is less tendency for the child to physically avoid the parent. Instead, they avoid a personal connection with the parent (Cassidy & Marvin, 1992; Main, 2000). Avoidant dyads are the other end of the spectrum from ambivalent/resistant dyads. There is little conflict between the parent and child. The avoidance in preschool-age children looks like avoiding rocking the boat. There is an avoidance of conflict rather than an avoidance of interaction.

The price the dyad pays for avoiding conflict is that they also avoid intimacy. Conflict, it turns out, is part of being in a secure relationship—especially with preschoolers who are beginning to explore the limits of their autonomy and independence. To the parent of a secure preschooler who is pushing boundaries all day, avoidant attachment may sound like a good alternative. However, it turns out that by missing out on the conflict, the parents of avoidant preschoolers are also missing out on the joy that comes with resolving conflict.

Often in avoidant dyads, the anger or anxiety the child feels at not getting their attachment needs met by their parent is expressed in other settings such as school or childcare. These children are often seen as mean by teachers, making it harder for the child to find alternative parent figures who might meet their attachment needs. The reason these children are seen as mean by teachers or childcare providers is that they apply their survival strategy when helping their peers cope with distress. This is the child who, when a peer is upset, may tease them. They have learned the lesson that distress is not to be tolerated. From their perspective, it is a tough world, and they want to impart this lesson to their peer. Needless to say, a child who responds to distress by heaping on more distress is seen as mean.

Prevalence of Avoidant Attachment

Ten to twenty percent of dyads in community samples exhibit avoidant attachment (Ainsworth et al., 1978; Moss et al., 2004). Approximately 10% of dyads referred to me for IoWA-PCIT exhibit an avoidant attachment.

Development of Avoidant Attachment

Lack of parental responsiveness to the child's distress is a major factor in the development of avoidant attachment (Ainsworth et al., 1978; Main, 2000). Parents of children with an avoidant attachment place greater emphasis on self-regulation and are concerned about spoiling children by being too responsive to crying and other indicators of distress. It is not that parents of children with avoidant attachment are less involved in their children's lives, it is the way they interact with their children. They are less likely to soothe their child when they are upset and more likely to encourage independence, self-regulation, and keeping a "stiff upper lip." This pattern is different from disorganized/avoidant attachment, where children are afraid to go to their parent for anything. Avoidant attachment, where the parent discourages what they perceive as neediness or vulnerability in the child, is subtler and less dramatic than disorganized/avoidant attachment, but it can still have a significant effect on the child's emotional regulation, relationship with the parent, and general view of relationships.

How Avoidant Attachment May Be Adaptive for the Child

The idea of avoidant attachment as a strategy to maintain proximity to the parent is a bit of a paradox. The child learns that in order to stay close enough to the parent that the parent is available in an emergency, the child must not be too demanding. I think of it like one of those "break glass in case of emergency" signs. It's reassuring to know it's there, but your threshold for declaring an emergency and breaking the glass is very high. This strategy has been described as deactivation of the attachment system. In other words, this strategy involves placing less emphasis on attachment needs, such as needing support from the parent when distressed.

The child in an avoidant attachment relationship with a parent has learned to rely on themselves and cope on their own. It is often easier to see how avoidant attachment is adaptive than it is to see how ambivalent/resistant attachment is adaptive. Being independent and being able to rely on oneself are important skills that are often valued.

How to Promote Secure Attachment in Avoidant Dyads

A key principle in helping avoidant dyads become more secure is helping the parent become more responsive to the child's distress. In van den Boom's study of her parent coaching intervention for irritable infants, coaching parents to be more responsive to their infant's attachment cues (including fussing and crying) at 6 months of age yielded huge dividends—cutting the rate of avoidant attachment by more than half (from 51% in the control group to 19% in the intervention group) (van den Boom, 1988, 1994). Child–Parent Psychotherapy (CPP), a dyadic intervention that helps parents recognize and respond to their child's attachment cues, also significantly reduces the rate of avoidant attachment in toddlers of depressed mothers (Toth et al., 2006). Thus, the research clearly shows that the path from avoidant to secure attachment involves helping parents become more sensitively responsive to distress.

The first step in coaching parents to become more responsive to their toddler's distress is for them to observe the cue. For example, the therapist might say, "I notice he is getting frustrated." The next step is to help the parent interpret the child's cue. One of the strategies used in CPP to help parents interpret their child's cue is "speaking for the child" (Lieberman & Van Horn, 2008; Toth et al., 2006). In other words, the therapist can suggest what the child might be trying to communicate to the parent—kind of like subtitles when you're watching a movie in a language you don't speak. For example, the therapist might say, "He seems to be thinking he could use some help calming down now." The therapist can also point out how the parent's response impacts the child. For example, the therapist might say, "He seems less frustrated since you moved closer and supported him."

Helping parents become more responsive to distress is more challenging when we are working with preschool-aged children as the child already has a well-established pattern of not showing vulnerability to their parent. By preschool age, young children in avoidant attachment relationships have learned a strategy of pretending (including to themselves) that they don't need their parent's support. Thus, it makes sense that once this pattern has become entrenched, the child expresses fewer episodes of distress to the parent and the parent has fewer opportunities to soothe their child's distress. It can feel a bit like a game of chicken when working with avoidant dyads where neither the parent nor the child wants to go first in being vulnerable. This means that, as therapists, it is often up to us to go first—suggesting the feelings we know, based on our deep understanding of attachment theory, that a child in an avoidant dyad is likely having.

Course of IoWA-PCIT with Avoidant Dyads

IoWA-PCIT is effective in reducing disruptive behavior in avoidant dyads. The biggest challenge is getting the parents in avoidant dyads to engage in treatment and participate in the parent coaching sessions. In my clinical experience, dyads with an avoidant attachment are the group most likely to drop out prior to the parent coaching sessions.

Working with avoidant dyads is also challenging because the avoidance has worked so well to maintain neutrality. I find myself reluctant to rock the boat when working with avoidant dyads. One of the things I like about a skill-based approach to working with avoidant attachment is that it provides a kind of scaffolding for the parent and child as they embark on the very tough work of letting their guard down with each other. Child-Directed Interaction (CDI) (described in Chap. 4) provides a type of rule book for how to be in relationship. As the parent becomes more adept at describing and reflecting, the child begins to let their guard down and trust that the parent is interested in who they are.

Praise can be a bit trickier in avoidant dyads. While, at their core, children in avoidant dyads want to be appreciated by their parents, they will sometimes reject the praise—doing the exact opposite of the behavior the parent has just praised. For example, a parent praises the child for coloring carefully and the child looks at the parent and scribbles on their paper. I have a couple of hypotheses about why avoidant children might respond negatively to praise at times. One is that praise is more evaluative than describing and reflecting. Since the focus of the relationship in avoidant dyads is on the child's independence and achievement, I think the child rejects the praise as a way to make the parent's opinion not matter—a protection against vulnerability. Another hypothesis is the child is concerned the praise will be followed by criticism and wants to beat the parent to the criticism by giving the parent something to criticize.

In avoidant dyads, the child and parent often do not appear to enjoy spending time together. In truth, I also struggle to enjoy spending time with avoidant dyads. The play in avoidant dyads can be somewhat boring compared to the imaginative play of more secure dyads. This is one of those situations where, as therapists, we need to set the stage and trust the child's inborn drive for play and attachment. In other words, we cannot "make" a child enjoy spending time with their parent. However, we can facilitate that enjoyment by providing a calm setting and an attentive parent.

Parent-Directed Interaction (PDI) (described in Chap. 5) tends to go fairly smoothly with avoidant dyads once the CDI phase has been completed. In my experience, one of the most difficult parts of PDI for children in an avoidant dyad is returning to play with their parent following a time-out from positive reinforcement. The child sometimes returns to a strategy of avoiding interaction or engaging in superficial interaction with the parent following a time-out for noncompliance with a command. When this happens, I coach the parent to describe their own play until the child is willing to play with them again. The child will eventually begin playing with the parent, giving the child an opportunity to repair by engaging in CDI. This opportunity to engage in repair following a rupture helps these dyads begin to build a new way of managing conflict.

It is my impression that the dyad often recognizes the limitations of their avoidant attachment strategy in the face of significant stress or trauma. It is as though these chinks in their avoidant armor provide the opportunity for interacting in a new way. The initial stress for many dyads with avoidant attachment is the stress of having to seek help from someone. It's important to remember that difficulty with being vulnerable and seeking help are at the core of the struggle in avoidant attachment. As therapists, we are used to parents seeking help and advice from us, so it's easy for us to forget what a big deal seeking help is for avoidant dyads. Thus, for avoidant dyads, the therapist acknowledging the effort to come in for treatment is especially important. Both the child and parent need to know you appreciate them coming to see you.

The Bottom Line

IoWA-PCIT is effective with dyads with avoidant attachment. When working with dyads with avoidant attachment, it is important to remember that seeking treatment and spending time together takes tremendous courage given their tendency to avoid vulnerability. Helping parents recognize and respond to distress is especially important when working with avoidant dyads. The CDI phase of IoWA-PCIT is particularly challenging for avoidant dyads as they learn to enjoy spending time together. During PDI, avoidant dyads learn to repair following rupture.

References

Ainsworth, M., Blehar, M., Waters, E., & Wall, S. (1978). *Patterns of attachment: A psychological study of the strange situation*. Erlbaum.

Cassidy, J., & Marvin, R. (1992). *Attachment Organization in Preschool Children: Procedures and coding manual*. University of Virginia.

Lieberman, A., & Van Horn, P. (2008). *Psychotherapy with infants and young children: Repairing the effects of stress and trauma on early attachment.* The Guilford Press.

Main, M. (2000). The organized categories of infant, child, and adult attachment: Flexible vs. inflexible attention under attachment-related stress. *Journal of the American Psychoanalytic Association, 48*, 1055–1096.

Moss, E., Cyr, C., & Dubois-Comtois, K. (2004). Attachment at early school age and developmental risk: Examining family contexts and behavior problems of controlling-caregiving, controlling-punitive, and behaviorally disorganized children. *Developmental Psychology, 40*(4), 519–532.

Toth, S., Rogosch, F., Manly, J., & Cicchetti, D. (2006). The efficacy of toddler-parent psychotherapy to reorganize attachment in the young offspring of mothers with major depressive disorder: A randomized preventive trial. *Journal of Consulting and Clinical Psychology, 74*, 1006–1016.

van den Boom, D. (1988). *Neonatal irritability and the development of attachment: Observation and intervention* (Dissertation). University of Leiden,

van den Boom, D. (1994). The influence of temperament and mothering on attachment and exploration: An experimental manipulation of sensitive responsiveness among lower-class mothers with irritable infants. *Child Development, 65*, 1457–1477.

Chapter 12
What Does Not Kill Me Makes Me Stronger: How to Tailor Coaching for Parents with Dismissing Attachment

This chapter discusses how to adapt parent coaching for parents who have a dismissing working model of attachment. Particular attention is paid to recognizing how the parent's dismissing attachment colors their perceptions of the child and the therapist and how to take this into account when coaching parents with dismissing attachment.

How to Recognize Dismissing Attachment

The parent working model of attachment associated with avoidant parent–child dyads is called dismissing attachment (George et al., 1984; Main, 2000). Individuals with a dismissing attachment working model place less emphasis on the importance of attachment relationships and more emphasis on self-reliance. One of the ways in which individuals with dismissing attachment dismiss the importance of early attachment relationships is by failing to remember negative early experiences or the negative impact of stressful early attachment experiences. Just as avoidant infants turn away from their parents when distressed, adults with dismissing attachment turn away from distressing early experiences.

Individuals with dismissing attachment often describe their childhood interactions with their parents as normal or even exceptional, for example, describing their parents as very loving and describing themselves as spoiled. However, they are unable to give any specific memories of their childhood relationships with their parents.

We get some hints about the parent's working model of attachment from watching their interactions with their child during the pretreatment assessment. Parents with dismissing attachment do not appear comfortable interacting with their child. It is not just that they don't appear to enjoy playing, they appear uncomfortable—like someone who does not have experience with children trying to make awkward small talk with a child.

Another source of information about the parent's working model of attachment is what they sound like—that is, how they communicate with us about their own needs and their child's needs. Research using the Adult Attachment Interview (AAI) (George et al., 1984; Main, 2000) provides an idea of the type of language individuals with a dismissing working model of attachment use when discussing their childhood attachment experiences with an interviewer. Individuals with dismissing attachment either devalue attachment and attachment experiences in an actively dismissive way or their descriptions of their attachment figures are positive or idealized.

The group of individuals with dismissing attachment who describe their childhood attachment experiences in extremely negative terms insist these experiences did not affect them. Both dismissing individuals who are overly positive about their parents and those who are devaluing avoid discussing—and perhaps feeling—the effect their attachment-related experiences have had on them. Just as babies avoid seeking proximity when distressed, the dismissing adults they grow into avoid expressing distress. By failing to admit to themselves that their parents failed to meet their attachment needs, individuals who idealize their parents are able to maintain the illusion that their parents would have met their attachment needs—if they had had those needs. Like the infants and young children in avoidant dyads described in Chap. 11, they deactivate their needs for attachment in order to stay in the relationship (Main, 2000).

Individuals who devalue attachment needs have not maintained the illusion that their parents met their attachment needs—instead, they devalue the needs themselves. When individuals with a dismissing working model of attachment admit to vulnerability or early difficult experiences in their childhoods, they often follow the description up with a positive wrap-up, some version of "What does not kill me makes me stronger" (Nietzsche, 1888).

How Dismissing Attachment May Be Adaptive

It is important to think about how aspects of dismissing attachment may be adaptive so we can understand the resistance we often face from dismissing parents to changing their way of interacting with their child. From the perspective of individuals with dismissing attachment, deactivation of the attachment system is a strategy that has worked well. Thus, they are reluctant to examine the ways it has not worked for them and is not working for their child. Also, because dismissing attachment is relatively prevalent in both the community (Bakermans-Kranenburg & van Ijzendoorn, 2009; Booth-LaForce & Roisman, 2014; Caspers et al., 2007) and amongst therapists (Talia et al., 2018), I find therapists tend to view dismissing attachment as more adaptive than preoccupied attachment.

It is clear how one of the core components of dismissing attachment—being self-reliant—may be an adaptive strategy. For individuals with dismissing attachment, the focus on overcoming challenges and not dwelling on difficult childhoods is an effective strategy for managing hardship. It is as though individuals with dismissing attachment are preparing their child for the harsh childhood they experienced, unaware that they are recreating a similarly harsh childhood by focusing on their child's self-reliance.

The ability to set aside feelings, another component of dismissing attachment, can also be an adaptive way of handling stress. In a crisis, being able to focus on taking action and addressing the crisis has definite short-term advantages.

Prevalence of Dismissing Attachment

Dismissing attachment is the second most prevalent type of attachment in community samples. Approximately one-third of individuals in community samples have a dismissing state of mind (Bakermans-Kranenburg & van Ijzendoorn, 2009; Booth-LaForce & Roisman, 2014; Caspers et al., 2007). A similar rate is found in parents participating in parent management training to address their child's disruptive behavior disorder (Routh et al., 1995), but the rate of dismissing attachment is significantly lower in parents participating in a preventive home-visiting intervention (Erickson et al., 1992). This is consistent with my clinical observation that dismissing parents tend to wait until problems are more severe to seek out help from a therapist. Dismissing attachment is the second most common type of attachment amongst therapists with 22% of therapists displaying this type of attachment (Talia et al., 2018).

Course of IoWA-PCIT with Dismissing Parents

Individuals with a dismissing attachment state of mind are less likely to seek out psychotherapy services or to ask for help from others. In a study we conducted with over 200 adults who had been adopted as infants, we found that individuals with dismissing working model of attachment were significantly less likely to have sought treatment for substance abuse, although their rates of substance abuse were comparable to individuals with preoccupied or earned secure attachment (Caspers et al., 2006). As noted in the chapter on avoidant attachment (Chap. 11), one of the keys to improving the child–parent relationship for avoidant dyads is helping the parent be more responsive to the child's distress and attachment cues. When coaching dismissing parents, it is important to keep in mind that what may seem obvious to us goes against their core strategy for being in relationship. Parents with dismissing attachment must learn to override their tendency to ignore distress.

The majority of parents I work with who have a dismissing working model of attachment feel coerced into treatment. Typically, they are seeking help for their child due to concerns by the school, the courts, or the child welfare system. Thus, my efforts to form a therapeutic alliance are hampered by their general tendency to not expect others to be helpful and their anger at feeling forced to meet with me.

As noted in the chapter on conducting an attachment-informed assessment (Chap. 3), forming a therapeutic relationship with parents begins at the initial evaluation. This is especially critical when working with parents with dismissing attachment. Just getting in the door is a huge achievement for these parents. They are willing to do it for the sake of their child. We need to remember and value that. Even though their willingness to come to treatment is often the result of a big nudge from the school or court system, they still had the choice of whether to comply with the demand to get treatment for them and their child. Since these parents often come to treatment with a chip on their shoulder, I have to remind myself to express my appreciation to them for coming to treatment.

The engage and teach session is also an important opportunity to form a therapeutic alliance with dismissing parents. Unlike secure and preoccupied parents, who value improving their relationship with their child, parents with a dismissing attachment are primarily focused on addressing their child's behavior problems. With dismissing parents, I tend to downplay the relationship aspects of the treatment during the engage and teach session. Instead, I focus on how IoWA-PCIT will help address the behavior problems that brought them to treatment. These are the parents most likely to express skepticism about a relationship-based approach. Rather than trying to convince them of the power of attachment, I emphasize how I will have their back during the coaching sessions. I describe how I will be able to see when their child misbehaves and help them respond to behavior problems in the moment. In other words, I describe a relationship where I will provide them with a safe haven during difficult interactions.

For individuals with a dismissing attachment state of mind, attending to their child's emotional needs is the most difficult aspect of the treatment. Thus, starting with Child-Directed Interaction (CDI) (described in Chap. 3), rather than a focus on discipline and self-reliance, is counterintuitive for dismissing parents. However, I find if we can get past their initial skepticism about CDI, the structure of CDI provides dismissing parents with specific ways of interacting with their child and makes them more comfortable with following their child's lead. Often, within a couple of sessions, they have put down their phone and are on the floor with their child. It typically takes several more sessions for them to become comfortable with attending to their own or their child's feelings, especially feelings of distress. One of the goals of the therapist is to attend to the parent's unmet needs, specifically their unmet need to express distress. Individuals with a dismissing state of mind do not make this easy. Research on the statements of such individuals during psychotherapy indicates they tend to cut off the therapist's attempts to attend to their feelings, usually by minimizing distress (Miller-Bottome et al., 2019; Talia et al., 2014).

When I talk with parents who have dismissing attachment state of mind about their own childhoods, they tend to downplay difficulties, describing themselves as spoiled and their childhoods as idyllic. It is only when details come out about their childhood as they begin to trust me that I learn that their childhoods have not been idyllic, and in what ways their emotional needs were not met during childhood.

Research indicates individuals with dismissing attachment are also more likely to use active distancing strategies with their significant others when sensitive topics are raised such as sighing or making sarcastic comments (Dozier, 2001). Navigating how to respond when parents sigh or make sarcastic comments to their children or us is challenging. It is important to recognize this as a defensive strategy. In other words, our natural reaction is to respond negatively to a parent sighing or making sarcastic comments. However, this is a way of protecting themselves from uncomfortable feelings. We have to realize that if we had subtitles during the interaction, the sigh or sarcasm means, "I'm feeling uncomfortable now so I'm trying to push you away." Then, instead of responding in kind, we can comment on what we suspect is going on with the parent—for example, "I can see this is challenging right now. I appreciate the way you are hanging in there with him."

During parent coaching, I am sensitive to moments when the parent may feel rejected by their child so I can offer conjectures about what the parent might be feeling. For example, when the child criticizes the parent's drawing ability, I might say something like, "Ouch. It is tough to be criticized by your child." I believe it is my ability to hold their feelings during these moments that allows them to begin to hold their child's tender feelings.

Parents with a dismissing state of mind tend to tune out their child's negative affect—just as they learned to tune out their own negative affect (Haft & Slade, 1989). The tendency to tune out both negative and positive affects in infant–parent interactions is seen in the physiological responses of pregnant women to video vignettes of infant–parent interactions (Ablow et al., 2013). In this research, pregnant women were shown brief video segments of a mother unable to soothe her crying infant and a mother playing contentedly with a baby while the researchers assessed their physiological response (heart rate, skin conductance, and respiratory sinus arrhythmia). The physiological responses of mothers with dismissing attachment indicated they found watching these videos aversive (Ablow et al., 2013). Thus, even before the birth of their child, dismissing parents have internalized, at a physiological level, the expectation that infant–parent interactions are uncomfortable, whether those interactions involve a crying or contented infant. This is consistent with my clinical observation that individuals with dismissing attachment often seem uncomfortable during interactions with their children.

Individuals with a dismissing state of mind are less likely to express distress to their therapist or ask for help (Talia et al., 2014). This makes our work somewhat more difficult than when working with parents with secure attachment since there are fewer openings to provide support and ideas about how to apply the IoWA-PCIT principles at home. Dismissing individuals are also less likely to express gratitude to their therapist (Talia et al., 2014). This lack of positive feedback is consistent with dismissing individuals' fear of vulnerability, but it can make it more challenging for therapists to feel the type of positive regard they feel for parents with secure attachment.

In Chap. 1, I talked about the impact of attachment priming on children. There is also a rich literature on the impact of attachment priming on adults. In a study on the impact of attachment priming on parents, parents were asked to "think about the person you can most depend on to be there to comfort you in times of trouble" (Jones et al., 2021). Dismissing parents who participated in this attachment prime had more positive attitudes toward their child. By communicating to parents that we are there for them, we are directly impacting their ability to be there for their child.

For dismissing parents, the most difficult aspect of Parent–Directed Interaction (PDI) (described in Chap. 5) is the sensitive part of providing sensitive discipline. We must stay alert to the possibility of the dismissing parent becoming too punitive during the PDI procedure or overusing PDI. These are the parents who are most likely to move too quickly to implementing PDI throughout the day that risks undermining their gains in CDI.

So far, I have been discussing how to coach a dismissing parent who has an avoidant relationship with their child, the most common combination. The next section focuses on coaching a dismissing parent who is not in an avoidant attachment relationship with their child.

Dismissing Parent in a Secure Relationship with Their Child

This has been one of the most surprising and heartening combinations in my work with parents and children. In these dyads, even though the parent feels uncomfortable with attending to the child's tender feelings, the parent has met the child's needs enough to develop a secure relationship. Because of our inborn desire and need for a healthy relationship with our parents, these children openly express their needs (e.g., "I'm sad," "I missed you," "I'm mad at you") in ways that might take years of individual psychotherapy for their dismissing parent to be able to do. Often, the parents in these dyads enter child–parent therapy with the vague idea that they need to be more like their own parents—more focused on discipline or not "spoiling" their child by responding to their distress, at the same time that these ideas make them vaguely uncomfortable.

The image that comes to mind when I think about these dyads is tender leaves poking through the ground in spring. I have the sense of needing to protect and nurture the secure attachment that is already there. When working with these dyads, I have had the unusual impression of the child being my co-therapist, helping the parent move into uncomfortable territory. As the child expresses their feelings to the parent, my job is to support the parent in moving into this uncomfortable territory. I let the parent know that their child's ability to directly communicate their attachment needs and feelings is a positive aspect of their relationship—even as I recognize it cannot always be easy to hear. In this way, I support the parent's emerging capacity for providing a haven of safety for the child.

Dismissing Parent in an Ambivalent/Resistant Relationship with Their Child

For these dyads, it is not just that the parent and child are speaking a different language—they are living on different planets. While the parent uses a strategy of deactivation in attachment relationships, the child uses a strategy of hyperactivation.

The more the parent ignores the child's distress and tries to "toughen up" the child, the more the child escalates and becomes needy and demanding.

With these dyads, my role is to teach both the parent and child a new language—the language of direct expression of their feelings and needs. An approach I have found especially helpful is having the parent model the ability to describe feelings for the child—for example, when the child is frustrated with a toy, asking the parent to model frustration, label their feeling by saying they are feeling frustrated, then model taking deep breaths to manage their frustration. I am also looking for opportunities to point out when the child labels their feelings—for example, saying they are mad instead of stomping their foot. Having the parent reflect the child's labeling of their feelings or praise the child for using their words to communicate their feelings serves two purposes. First, the child has the experience of their parent recognizing and responding to the child's attachment cues. Second, the parent has the experience of feelings being something that can be communicated without being overwhelming. When working with this combination, it is important to be patient with yourself, the parent, and the child. It takes a while to learn a new language.

The Bottom Line

When working with parents with dismissing attachment, we have the opportunity to help them move from deactivation of the attachment system to activation of the attachment system. In other words, we are able to help the parent learn to be more vulnerable and open in their relationship with their child and their relationship with us. Child-Directed Interaction (CDI) is especially important for parents with dismissing attachment. It provides them with the skills to develop a more positive relationship with their child and feel more comfortable interacting with their child.

References

Ablow, J., Marks, A., Feldman, S., & Huffman, L. (2013). Associations between first-time expectant women's representations of attachment and their physiological reactivity to infant cry. *Child Development, 84*(4), 1373–1391.

Bakermans-Kranenburg, M., & van Ijzendoorn, M. (2009). The first 10,000 adult attachment interviews: Distributions of adult attachment representations in clinical and non-clinical groups. *Attachment & Human Development, 11*(3), 223–263.

Booth-LaForce, C., & Roisman, G. (2014). The adult attachment interview: Psychometrics, stability and change from infancy and developmental origins. *Monographs of the Society for Research in Child Development, 79*(3), 1–185.

Caspers, K. M., Yucuis, R., Troutman, B., Arndt, S., & Langbehn, D. (2007). A sibling adoption study of adult attachment: The influence of shared environment on attachment state of mind. *Attachment & Human Development, 9*(4), 375–391.

Caspers, K. M., Yucuis, R., Troutman, B., & Spinks, R. (2006). Attachment as an organizer of behavior: Implications for substance abuse problems and willingness to seek treatment. *Substance Abuse Treatment, Prevention, and Policy, 1*, 32.

Dozier, M. (2001). The challenge of treatment for clients with dismissing state of mind. *Attachment & Human Development, 3*(1), 62–76.

Erickson, M., Korfmacher, J., & Egeland, B. (1992). Attachments past and present: Implications for therapeutic intervention with mother-infant dyads. *Development and Psychopathology, 4*, 495–507.

George, C., Kaplan, N., & Main, M. (1984). *Adult attachment interview*. University of California.

Haft, W., & Slade, A. (1989). Affect attunement and maternal attachment: A pilot study. *Infant Mental Health Journal, 10*(3), 157–172.

Jones, J., Stern, J., Fitter, M., Mikulincer, M., Shaver, P., & Cassidy, J. (2021). Attachment and attitudes toward children: Effects of security priming in parents and non-parents. *Attachment & Human Development., 24*(2), 147–168.

Main, M. (2000). The organized categories of infant, child, and adult attachment: Flexible vs. inflexible attention under attachment-related stress. *Journal of the American Psychoanalytic Association, 48*, 1055–1096.

Miller-Bottome, M., Talia, A., Eubanks, C., Safran, J., & Muran, J. (2019). Secure in-session attachment predicts rupture resolution: Negotiating a secure base. *Psychoanalytic Psychology, 36*(2), 132–138.

Nietzsche, F. (1888). *Twilight of the idols or how to philosophize with a hammer*. Penguin Classics.

Routh, C., Hill, J., Steele, H., Elliott, C., & Dewey, M. (1995). Maternal attachment status, psychosocial stressors and problem behaviour: Follow-up after parent training courses for conduct disorder. *Journal of Child Psychology and Psychiatry, 36*(7), 1179–1198.

Talia, A., Daniel, S., Miller-Bottome, M., Brambilla, D., Miccoli, D., Safran, J., & Lingiardi, V. (2014). AAI predicts patients' in-session interpersonal behavior and discourse: A "move to the level of the relation" for attachment-informed psychotherapy research. *Attachment & Human Development, 16*(2), 192–209.

Talia, A., Muzi, L., Lingiardi, V., & Taubner, S. (2018). How to be a secure base: therapists' attachment representations and their link to attunement in psychotherapy. *Attachment & Human Development., 22*(2), 189–206.

Chapter 13
Attachment Anxiety: How to Tailor Coaching for Dyads with Disorganized and Controlling Attachment

This chapter discusses the challenges of working with behaviorally disorganized and controlling child–parent dyads. I discuss the role of loss and trauma in the development of disorganized and controlling attachment. I describe how to address the emotional and behavioral problems of children in disorganized and controlling dyads using attachment-informed parent coaching.

This chapter deals with the dark side of attachment—the disorganizing impact of loss and trauma. It is the other side of the coin—the powerful impact of loss and developmental trauma is built into the powerful importance of attachment. You cannot understand attachment without understanding what happens when a young child experiences the loss of an attachment figure—and you cannot understand disorganized and controlling attachment relationships without understanding the extreme lengths individuals will go to in order to avoid losing the connection with an attachment figure. We have to look at the darkness of loss in order to fully understand the power of attachment.

When I look at the history of attachment theory, it seems inextricably tied with an effort to understand the impact of separation and loss. Notably, in Bowlby's trilogy laying out the tenets of attachment theory, the first volume is titled *Attachment* (Bowlby, 1969), the second volume is titled *Separation* (Bowlby, 1973), and the third volume is titled *Loss* (Bowlby, 1980). In Mary Ainsworth's initial observational study of mother–infant interaction, she sought to understand attachment by understanding what happened to infants when they were separated from their mothers for weaning—a practice she had been told (incorrectly) was common amongst the Ugandan (Ainsworth, 1967). And when Mary Ainsworth developed her standardized assessment of attachment, the Strange Situation Procedure, it included brief separations from the parent (Ainsworth et al., 1978). It is as though to truly understand the power of attachment we need to understand the impact of separation and loss.

Role of Loss in Disorganized Attachment

As noted in Chap. 1, the contributions of James and Joyce Robertson are especially important for understanding how the loss of a parent impacts young children (Robertson & Robertson, 1989). James and Joyce Robertson worked in the Hampstead nurseries founded by Anna Freud and Dorothy Burlingham to care for young children separated from their parents during World War II. Following the war, James and Joyce Robertson continued to study the impact of being separated from a parent on young children. The Robertsons vividly describe the withdrawal, irritability, anger, and aggression that occur when young children are separated from their parents (Robertson & Robertson, 1989). James Robertson also made a series of films showing the impact of separation on young children. When I show these films during workshops, the sadness and anger in the room is palpable as we watch young children exhibit protest, despair, and detachment. James and Joyce Robertson (1989) also examined the role of substitute parents in helping young children cope with separation and loss. Specifically, young children had the most difficulty coping with separation when placed in a group setting where they did not have a consistent caregiver to help them cope with their grief and anxiety about their separation from their parent. In order to better understand how they might mitigate the impact of separation, the Robertsons served as foster parents for a number of young children. The importance of the Robertsons' observations is twofold. First, they document the distress of young children to being separated from their parents. Second, they provide hope for ameliorating the negative impact of separation, noting how the availability of a responsive substitute parent can help children cope with separation (Robertson & Robertson, 1989).

Winnicott, a pediatrician and psychoanalyst who also witnessed firsthand the impact of loss on young children during World War II, writes movingly of the disorganizing experience of losing a parent, even briefly, for young children in the passage below (Winnicott, 1987):

> If left for too long (hours, minutes) without familiar and human contact they have experiences which we can only describe by such words as:
>
> going to pieces
> falling for ever
> dying and dying and dying
> losing all vestige of hope of the renewal of contacts.

Winnicott's (1987) language evokes the visceral experience for infants and young children of the terrible truth that they are utterly dependent on others for their survival. His description makes clear why young children may develop a disorganized attachment when their parents are absent—either physically or psychologically.

In previous chapters on patterns of attachment, I described what the pattern of attachment looked like before discussing what factors contributed to the pattern. I wanted to make this chapter follow the same format, but it just wouldn't—it is just not possible to wrap your head around disorganized attachment without starting with loss and trauma. However, my fear is that readers will come away with the assumption that every time they see disorganization in an attachment relationship, they need to identify the loss or trauma. This is certainly not the case. There are times when we are unable to identify loss or trauma—or even to know whether there has been loss or trauma in the life of the child. Disorganized attachment can result from unresolved trauma in the life of the parent that may not be obvious to the therapist. Disorganized attachment can also result from the cumulative stress in the lives of some of our young patients rather than a specific loss or trauma.

Role of Parents' Frightening Behavior in Disorganized/Disoriented Attachment

Parents exhibiting frightening behavior toward their child are associated with disorganized attachment. One author describes this as "a confusing cocktail of tenderness and terror" (Marino, 2015). In the organized patterns of attachment, there is some level of predictability that allows the child to develop a strategy for getting their attachment needs met. In disorganized attachment, this is not possible because while the parent provides a safe haven at times, they can also be the source of the anxiety. Because the parent is the source of the anxiety, the child is faced with a dilemma that cannot be resolved. The person they go to for comfort is also the source of their fear.

Role of Parents' Frightened Behavior in Disorganized/Disoriented Attachment

Some parents appear frightened of their child. This frightened behavior can be exhibited nonverbally. For example, the parent may pull back from the child or exhibit a sharp intake of breath—as though they have seen a wild animal or large imposing human rather than the small vulnerable human we are seeing. Parents can also communicate to their child that they are frightened of them through their verbalizations. For example, the parent may sound like they are pleading with the child. The content of the speech may be coded as commands or negative talk in the Dyadic Parent–Child Interaction Coding System (DPICS) (Eyberg et al., 2013) we use in IoWA-PCIT. However, the tone in which the command (e.g., "Please be careful") or the negative talk ("Please stop hitting me") is delivered sounds more like a child pleading with a parent than a parent communicating with a child.

A parent who is frightened of their child can be as disorganizing as a parent who frightens their child. It is not possible for the child to use a parent as a safe haven when they become distressed when the parent is more distressed or anxious than the child. In addition, parents who are frightened of their child are often too frightened to set limits on their child's behavior. So, in dyads where the parent is frightened of the child the child lacks the predictability and reassurance that comes with appropriate boundaries.

How to Recognize Disorganized/Disoriented Attachment

During the Strange Situation Procedure, disorganized/disoriented attachment may appear in the briefest of moments. In the nomenclature used to describe attachment relationships, dyads are given a secondary classification that describes the underlying pattern of attachment when the primary attachment classification is disorganized. The combination I have the most difficulty getting my head around is disorganized/secure. Disorganized/secure has also been described as disorganized moving toward (Lyons-Ruth & Spielman, 2004)—an apt description of what you see in the Strange Situation Procedure with these dyads. You see a baby who is going toward their parent to get their attachment needs met in a way that is typical of secure dyads—that is, moving toward the mother when distressed, greeting the mother when she returns. However, this typical secure behavior is mixed with anxiety and fear. These are interpreted as indications the baby is unable to reliably use the mother as a safe haven—pausing briefly with a dazed expression before moving toward the mother, freezing for 30 seconds before moving toward the mother, or showing increased anxiety when the mother returns after the separation by twirling their hair or sucking their thumb.

How to Recognize Disorganized/Controlling Attachment

There is a subset of disorganized attachment called controlling attachment. In disorganized/controlling attachment, the core aspect of the attachment relationship is the child's controlling behavior toward the parent. This controlling behavior is especially prevalent when the attachment system is activated—as it is following a separation. I have struggled with this nomenclature as controlling attachment relationships do not appear disorganized—they actually appear rigid and overly controlled. The disorganization describes the child's experience—that is, the concomitant anxiety associated with disorganized attachment. However, the controlling behavior describes what we see—the behavioral response to anxiety. Presumably, the child copes with their internal disorganization and anxiety within the attachment relationship by controlling the attachment relationship. Of course, all children try to control their environment, including their parents, in some way. Controlling attachment relationships have a different quality than young children's typical attempts to control their parents. In controlling attachment, the child is in control of the relationship. There is a profound role reversal in these relationships where the child has become the parent and the parent has become the child.

There are two types of controlling attachment relationships: controlling–punitive and controlling–caregiving. Children who have a controlling–punitive relationship manage their relationship with their parent by telling them what to do when their attachment needs are activated. After a brief separation from their parent, these preschoolers sound like an angry drill sergeant—telling the parent where to sit, what to do, and rejecting any attempts from the parent to engage with them following the separation. These are difficult interactions to watch. It would be difficult to watch a parent treat a child this way, but it is somehow even more chilling to watch a child treat a parent this way. It is very difficult for both the parent and the therapist to perceive the child as a child during these moments.

Controlling–caregiving is more subtle. When the parent returns after a brief separation, the child is *extremely* happy to see them. The greeting goes way beyond the casual relaxed pleasure seen in secure dyads—it is almost like a grotesque stereotype of that greeting. The child may exhibit what is referred to in the attachment literature as an "overbright" smile (Cassidy & Marvin, 1992). Perhaps it is the sensitivity of attachment researchers to the underlying attachment needs and anxiety being covered up by this greeting that keep them from describing it the way it feels which is fake. There is a lack of genuineness in the greeting that indicates the child is appeasing the parent rather than being truly happy for the parent's return. Another striking aspect of children in controlling–caregiving relationships with their parents is their willingness to set aside their own needs for acknowledgment by their parents in order meet their parent's needs. Interactions feel like a zero-sum game, and it is important that the parent always wins. The child makes sure that the parent's drawing is better than their drawing or that the parent wins at Candyland. It is hard to describe just how exhausting it is for a young child to be continually making themself smaller in order to remain in an attachment relationship with their parent. While the emotional reaction to controlling–punitive is immediate and overwhelming for most therapists, the reaction to controlling–caregiving is more subtle. The best way I can describe my reaction to these dyads is that it feels a bit creepy. Something is off but it is difficult to put my finger on it. The helpfulness on the part of the child doesn't feel genuine. There is a forced and anxious quality to their need to be so helpful to their parent. It also feels a bit sad.

Development of Controlling Attachment

We know that some, but not all, disorganized attachment relationships evolve into controlling attachment relationships as children get older. When trying to explain why some young children with disorganized attachment go on to develop controlling attachment, I turn again to the eloquent words of Winnicott, who is so good at putting himself into the mind of a baby: "A certain proportion of babies have experienced environmental failure while dependence was a fact, and then, in varying degrees, there is damage done, damage that can be difficult to repair. At best the baby growing into a child and an adult carries round a buried memory of a disaster that happened to the self, and much time and energy are spent in organizing life so that such pain may not be experienced again" (Winnicott, 1987).

Rather than experience that "falling into the abyss" (Winnicott, 1987) that occurs when babies are unable to rely on a parent to help them manage their anxiety, young children develop a strategy of controlling their parent. It is not the same as truly getting their attachment needs met, but it is a strategy that allows them to be in relationship and avoid the awful experience of anxiety that follows them from infancy. Perhaps it is because I sense how deeply these young children want to be in relationship that I have a strong reaction when others suggest children who are trying to control their parents are unattached.

Recent research on the specific parent behaviors associated with controlling–punitive and controlling–caregiving attachment can help us understand the specific parent behaviors we need to address when working with these dyads (Lecompte et al., 2021). Controlling–caregiving behaviors are associated with less maternal-sensitive responsiveness (Lecompte et al., 2021). In other words, when the parent fails to respond sensitively to the child's attachment signals, the child may become the parent's caregiver—putting the parent's needs ahead of their own in order to be in relationship with the parent. Controlling–punitive behaviors are associated with less maternal structuring (Lecompte et al., 2021). That is, when the parent fails to provide the child with the necessary structure and support the child becomes the parent— structuring the relationship by taking charge and giving the parent commands.

How Disorganized/Disoriented Attachment May Be Adaptive for the Child

Disorganized/disoriented attachment indicates a breakdown in attachment strategy. It is adaptive in the sense that disorganized/disoriented attachment, that is, the lack of a strategy, is actually the only possible strategy when consistently seeking support from a parent is not possible—either due to the loss of the parent or due to the parent provoking anxiety.

Disorganized/disoriented attachment reflects the flight or freeze response to stress when the child is faced with the ongoing stress of a parent who is frightened or frightening. The breakdown in attachment strategy seen in disorganized/disoriented attachment is adaptive in the sense it allows the child to be in relationship with an unavailable or maltreating parent with the only strategies available to a young child. That is, the child can escape by fleeing from the parent or cautiously seeking contact with the parent, even as their biological predisposition is to go to the parent for comfort. Or the child can escape by freezing—momentarily avoiding the stress associated with being scared and not being able to take this anxiety to a parent.

How Controlling Attachment May Be Adaptive for the Child

I think of controlling attachment as an adaptive solution to a maladaptive situation. In a dyad in which a parent is unpredictable, frightening, and/or frightened, it makes sense for the child to try to control the parent. There may be short-term benefits to coping with anxiety about the availability of the parent by becoming the caregiver for the parent (Moss et al., 2004). Specifically, controlling–caregiving may help a child cope with a parent's unresolved trauma or depression in the short term, providing the child with a way to be in relationship with a caregiver who is struggling with their own emotional needs. However, there may be long-term consequences to needing to always be the caregiver in the relationship. Ignoring their own needs may affect the child's ability to function effectively in peer relationships. The short-term benefits of controlling–punitive attachment are less obvious. The role reversal of becoming the parent is a way for the child to provide the structure that is lacking in the relationship.

Prevalence of Disorganized/Disoriented Attachment

In community samples, the rate of disorganized/disoriented attachment is approximately 15% (Greenberg et al., 1991; Speltz et al., 1990, 1999; van Ijzendoorn et al., 1999). Rates are higher in clinical and maltreatment samples (Toth et al., 2006). Among dyads with a clinically depressed mother, 30–40% exhibit disorganized/disoriented attachment (Toth et al., 2006; Troutman & Momany, 2012). Approximately 40% of preschoolers referred for disruptive behavior exhibit disorganized/disoriented attachment (Greenberg et al., 1991; Speltz et al., 1990, 1999). Approximately half of the young children referred for services following an investigation of maltreatment exhibit a disorganized/disoriented attachment (Bernard et al., 2012; Moss et al., 2011). Approximately 20% of dyads referred to me for IoWA-PCIT exhibit a disorganized/disoriented attachment.

Prevalence of Controlling Attachment

About 5% of dyads in community samples exhibit the controlling subtype of disorganized/disoriented attachment (Moss et al., 2004). In my clinical experience, approximately 5% of dyads referred to me for IoWA-PCIT exhibit the controlling subtype of disorganized/disoriented attachment. Although the rate of controlling attachment is relatively low in dyads referred to me, there are some elements of controlling attachment (i.e., some indicators of controlling–punitive and/or controlling–caregiving attachment) in approximately 40% of the dyads evaluated prior to IoWA-PCIT. In other words, while it is relatively rare for controlling attachment to be the primary feature of the relationship, it is relatively common for the children referred to me for IoWA-PCIT to engage in efforts to control or manage their parent.

Course of IoWA-PCIT with Disorganized/Disoriented and Controlling Attachment Relationships

IoWA-PCIT is a trauma-informed intervention that acknowledges the terrible ways in which children have had to adapt to terrible circumstances. It is a sad, hard truth that we cannot erase the terrible events that have affected some of the families we see for therapy. We need to start with a recognition of our limitations—our inability to "undo" the loss or trauma by returning the child to a previous developmental stage. Instead, our starting point is improving the child's current relationships with parents and doing whatever we can to reduce the child's ongoing exposure to adverse experiences.

Young children need relationships with parents to survive and thrive. Thus, the loss of a parent can be particularly disorganizing for young children. When a young child has lost a parent, the focus of the therapy is helping the child develop an organized secure attachment relationship with another parent. Sometimes, this involves focusing on the relationship with the surviving parent who is experiencing their own loss. At other times, the loss results in the child developing a new parental relationship. I have found Child-Directed Interaction (CDI) helpful in helping the child forge a new parental relationship or improve an existing parental relationship.

Interventions such as IoWA-PCIT that target the child–parent relationship address the impact of early trauma because the most devastating types of early trauma are those that involve traumatic relationships with parents. Our goal is to free children from the strategies they have had to use in order to cope with loss, frightening parents, and or frightened parents, and help them find new ways of being in relationship. This goal obviously involves the assumption that the frightening or frightened parent is making changes as well. To be perfectly honest, this is probably the assumption I struggle with the most when working with disorganized and controlling dyads. I have learned to trust the wisdom of children to understand when their parent has made the changes necessary for the child to be able to interact with their parent in new, more secure ways. The work with parents necessary to allow children to make these changes will be discussed in Chap. 14 on unresolved attachment in parents.

When working with disorganized and controlling dyads, I have several potential tasks—helping the child tolerate increasing levels of anxiety and dysregulation, addressing the behavior problems, helping the child trust attachment relationships following a loss, addressing the parent's frightening or fearful behavior, and helping the child learn an organized strategy for getting their attachment needs met. These are the dyads where I feel most strongly about trying to get the parent into their own individual treatment. I have found without this in place it is difficult to make sustained progress with dyads with disorganized attachment. In Chap. 14, I discuss the treatment approaches that seem to be especially helpful for parents with unresolved attachment.

In work with disorganized and controlling attachment, one of the most important goals is to reduce the parent's frightening or frightened behavior during interactions with the child—the specific behaviors associated with disorganized attachment. Keeping the IoWA-PCIT room a safe place where neither the child nor the parent engages in dangerous or destructive behavior is part of how we begin to reduce the risk for disorganized attachment.

Lack of recognition by a parent is at the heart of disorganized attachment. In other words, it is the parent's inability to imagine their child's experience and put themselves in their child's shoes that contributes to the parent behaving in ways that fail to recognize the child's needs. Because lack of recognition is such a core component of disorganized attachment, I find that active ignore and time-out from positive reinforcement can be especially distressing for dyads with a disorganized attachment. In disorganized dyads, the child can become so anxious about the parent's lack of attention that they are unable to tolerate the active ignore and time-out—reacting with a spiral of increasing anxiety. This seems to be especially true when working with dyads where there is a controlling–caregiving or controlling–punitive strategy. Because the controlling strategy works so well at managing their anxiety and their parent's behavior, the child is loath to give it up.

The child's experience with their parent, and by extension, their blueprint for interactions with other adults, also means they are unlikely to trust the therapist and the therapist's motives for taking away the controlling strategy that works so well for them. The most important tenet for working with dyads where disorganization and controlling are prevalent is to pay attention to the indicators of anxiety without being overwhelmed by them. A child who has a complete meltdown during an active ignore means you need to modify how you do an active ignore—not that you need to completely change your treatment approach.

The experience of coaching disorganized and controlling dyads is much like the experience of being in a disorganized or controlling attachment relationship. Everything seems to be going along swimmingly when out of the blue there is a disaster. Because of the sudden affective shifts that occur in disorganized and controlling dyads, it is difficult to predict when the change is going to occur. This can leave therapists feeling unsettled and anxious when working with disorganized and controlling dyads.

Because anxiety and intense affect is such a feature of these dyads, it is important that therapists recognize their own typical ways of responding to stress and anxiety—not necessarily to prevent their usual, very human responses to stress but in order to recognize when they have become caught in the "disorganized spiral" (Powell et al., 2014) so they can address their own anxiety. The disorganized spiral refers to the way in which the dyad's uncontained anxiety can spread to the therapist (Powell et al., 2014). In addition to recognizing their typical ways of responding to stress and anxiety, it is important that therapists have "go to" strategies that work for them for managing their anxiety. In Chap. 18, I discuss one of my go to strategies—taking a dance break. Walking to get a cup of coffee or talking with a colleague are also stress relievers for me. Whatever strategy I choose, I've learned the importance of taking just a couple of minutes for myself before appointments with disorganized dyads so that I'm less likely to become caught up in their anxiety and better able to help them contain it.

One of the striking aspects of disorganized and controlling dyads is the way in which relatively typical events suddenly turn into something different. I think it is part of the reason working with these dyads can be so unsettling. Something feels weird or off in the child and parent's reaction—a sensation as therapists that we hate to admit experiencing. It is not unusual for young children to accidentally hurt themselves during IoWA-PCIT sessions. We are working with young, impulsive, sometimes reckless individuals who are still figuring out how to find their way in the physical world. Children bump their heads, trip when running, dance too wildly, and careen into the wall. In most dyads, the parent responds by checking to see if the child is okay, perhaps followed by a brief cuddle. In disorganized dyads, the reaction is of an entirely different sort. For example, after the child bumps his head, the parent laughs and then criticizes him for not being more careful. The child may laugh along with the parent or suddenly become intensely angry.

When parents and children go off script like this, the therapist's anxiety may cause the therapist to freeze—standing behind the mirror stunned at what happened. It is difficult to keep the child in mind in these moments. However, holding the child in mind is the most important thing we can do in that moment. We need to take a deep breath and ask the parent the question that is part of the usual script when children get hurt—that is, "Is he okay?" We can then describe what we saw—"Wow—it sounded like he really hit his head hard." We might even need to suggest a new way of responding to the parent such as "Can you ask him if he is okay?" In these moments, we also need to keep the parent in mind. We need to remember that these types of stressful situations are the ones most likely to evoke their overlearned ways of responding to stress or anxiety. We can acknowledge the anxiety by saying things like "It's so hard when children hurt themselves. Hard on them and hard on you." We may also need to help them understand their child's reaction. "I know he is laughing but I think that scared him a little." Or, "I know he seems angry at you right now. I think he is upset because he hurt himself."

The Bottom Line

IoWA-PCIT is effective at reducing disruptive behavior and beginning to heal the impact of early attachment trauma. When coaching parents of children in disorganized and controlling attachment relationships with their parent, the therapist must stay attuned to managing and reducing any anxiety. This includes attending to and addressing their own anxiety to prevent getting caught up in the disorganized spiral that is often a feature of working with these dyads. The therapist must also attend to frightening and frightened parent behaviors that contribute to disorganized and controlling behavior in child–parent interactions. Finally, the therapist must attend to recognizing and responding to indications the child is becoming anxious, remembering that when you see controlling behavior it is an indication of anxiety.

During CDI, the child begins to have the experience they missed earlier in their life—the experience of a sensitively responsive parent who recognizes their attachment needs and responds. For children in disorganized attachment relationships, the experience of being seen, heard, and acknowledged is a powerful experience. During PDI, the child begins to have the experience of effective limit-setting. That is, they learn to follow their parent's directions in a calm, predictable environment where their parent is neither frightened of them nor frightening.

References

Ainsworth, M. (1967). *Infancy in Uganda*. Johns Hopkins Press.
Ainsworth, M., Blehar, M., Waters, E., & Wall, S. (1978). *Patterns of attachment: A psychological study of the strange situation*. Erlbaum.
Bernard, K., Dozier, M., Bick, J., Lewis-Morrarty, E., Lindhiem, O., & Carlson, E. (2012). Enhancing attachment organization among maltreated children: Results of a randomized clinical trial. *Child Development, 83*(2), 623–636.
Bowlby, J. (1969). *Attachment and loss. Vol 1: Attachment*. Basic Books.
Bowlby, J. (1973). *Separation: Anxiety and anger*. Basic Books.
Bowlby, J. (1980). *Loss: Sadness and depression*. Basic Books.
Cassidy, J., & Marvin, R. (1992). *Attachment Organization in Preschool Children: Procedures and coding manual*. University of Virginia.
Eyberg, S., Nelson, M., Ginn, N., Bhuiyan, N., & Boggs, S. (2013). *Dyadic parent-child interaction coding system (DPICS): Comprehensive manual for research and training*. PCIT International, Inc..
Greenberg, M., Speltz, M., DeKlyen, M., & Endriga, M. (1991). Attachment security in preschoolers with and without externalizing behavior problems: A replication. *Development and Psychopathology, 3*, 413–430.
Lecompte, V., Robins, S., King, L., Solomonova, E., Khan, N., Moss, E., … Zelkowitz, P. (2021). Examining the role of mother-child interactions and DNA methylation of the oxytocin receptor gene in understanding child controlling attachment behaviors. *Attachment & Human Development, 23*(1), 37–55.
Lyons-Ruth, K., & Spielman, E. (2004). Disorganized infant attachment strategies and helpless-fearful profiles of parenting: Integrating attachment research with clinical intervention. *Infant Mental Health Journal, 25*(4), 318–335.
Marino, G. (2015). The long conversation. *The New York Times*. June 2.
Moss, E., Cyr, C., & Dubois-Comtois, K. (2004). Attachment at early school age and developmental risk: Examining family contexts and behavior problems of controlling-caregiving, controlling-punitive, and behaviorally disorganized children. *Developmental Psychology, 40*(4), 519–532.
Moss, E., Dubois-Comtois, K., Cyr, C., St-Laurent, D., & Bernier, A. (2011). Efficacy of a home-visiting intervention aimed at improving maternal sensitivity, child attachment, and behavioral outcomes for maltreated children: A randomized control trial. *Development and Psychopathology, 23*, 195–210.
Powell, B., Cooper, G., Hoffman, K., & Marvin, R. (2014). *The circle of security intervention: Enhancing attachment in early parent-child relationships*. The Guilford Press.
Robertson, J., & Robertson, J. (1989). *Separation and the very young*. Free Association Books.

Speltz, M., DeKlyen, M., & Greenberg, M. (1999). Attachment in boys with early onset conduct problems. *Development and Psychopathology, 11*, 269–285.

Speltz, M., Greenberg, M., & DeKlyen, M. (1990). Attachment in preschoolers with disruptive behavior: A comparison of clinic-referred and nonproblem children. *Development and Psychopathology, 2*, 31–46.

Toth, S., Rogosch, F., Manly, J., & Cicchetti, D. (2006). The efficacy of toddler-parent psychotherapy to reorganize attachment in the young offspring of mothers with major depressive disorder: A randomized preventive trial. *Journal of Consulting and Clinical Psychology, 74*, 1006–1016.

Troutman, B., & Momany, A. (2012). Use of selective serotonin reuptake inhibitors during pregnancy and disorganised infant-mother attachment. *Journal of Reproductive and Infant Psychology, 30*(3), 261–277.

van Ijzendoorn, M., Schungel, C., & Bakermans-Kranenburg, M. J. (1999). Disorganized attachment in early childhood: Meta-analysis of precursors, concomitants, and sequelae. *Development and Psychopathology, 11*, 225–249.

Winnicott, D. W. (1987). *Babies and their mothers*. Addison-Wesley Publishing Company, Inc.

Chapter 14
Ghosts in the Playroom: How to Tailor Coaching for Parents with Unresolved Attachment Loss or Trauma

This chapter discusses how to adapt parent coaching for parents with unresolved attachment associated with loss and/or trauma. I describe how to recognize unresolved attachment loss or trauma and the importance of keeping the parent in mind when coaching a parent with their own attachment trauma. I discuss additional interventions that may be useful to parents with unresolved trauma and how to incorporate aspects of those interventions into IoWA-PCIT coaching.

How to Recognize Unresolved Attachment Loss or Trauma

I was googling Beatrice Beebe, one of my favorite attachment researchers, to see if she was offering any workshops on attachment when I came across an article written by Gordon Marino about his long-term psychotherapy with Beatrice Beebe. When describing his reasons for seeking psychotherapy, he states, "When the froth of my inner life came to a boil, I had no way of calming myself down and would invariably transform inner theater into street theater" (Marino, 2015).

It's the best description I've read of the experience of coaching parents with unresolved attachment. When coaching parents with unresolved attachment, I see sudden shifts of affect during stressful moments. I've seen parents suddenly freeze, glare at their child, begin yelling at their child, or begin pleading with their child. There is a quality to the interaction that suggests the parent is experiencing something other than what's happening with the child in the room—that in their mind the parent is pleading with or arguing with someone from their past.

On the Adult Attachment Interview (AAI) (George et al., 1984; Main, 2000), unresolved loss or trauma is revealed through specific ways of discussing the loss or trauma. Indicators include lapses where the individual seems to lose their train of thought (presumably brief moments of dissociation), blaming themselves for the loss or trauma, and talking about someone who is deceased as though they are still alive.

Development of Unresolved Attachment

Loss of an attachment figure or trauma is a necessary prerequisite for a parent to exhibit unresolved attachment. However, it is important to keep in mind that not everyone who experiences loss or trauma has unresolved attachment. It is a painful truth that it is difficult to get through childhood without experiencing some loss of an attachment figure.

In a study of adults who were adopted as infants, we found that the vast majority (97%) had experienced loss or trauma (Caspers et al., 2007). We also found that the vast majority of those who had experienced loss or trauma (71%) had reached some resolution of this loss or trauma, as assessed by the AAI (Caspers et al., 2007). In other words, for most of the individuals who had experienced loss or trauma, they were able to describe the experience in a contained way, perhaps with great sadness or anger but without blaming themselves or becoming confused. We found some evidence that individuals who are genetically predisposed to anxiety and depression are more likely to exhibit unresolved attachment (Caspers et al., 2009).

How Unresolved Attachment May Be Adaptive

Like disorganized attachment, unresolved attachment is adaptive in that it is a way of coping with a seemingly unsolvable dilemma. Adopting the characteristics typical of people with unresolved attachment avoids the pain of loss and abuse in the only way that feels possible when faced with an unsolvable dilemma. For example, one characteristic of individuals with unresolved attachment is blaming themselves for loss or maltreatment by a parent. Although there are certainly negative consequences to this self-blame, it protects the individual from recognizing the vulnerability and lack of control they experienced as a vulnerable young child. Another characteristic is dissociation, what has been referred to as "the escape when there is no escape" (Putnam, 1992).

Interventions Associated with Resolution of Unresolved Attachment

When thinking about coaching parents with unresolved attachment, it is helpful to be informed about some of the interventions that may be useful to individuals with unresolved attachment. I'm not suggesting that we're treating the parent's unresolved attachment during parent coaching, but it is useful to think about how we can support the parent's mental health and attachment needs during parent coaching.

The majority of parents I coach who have unresolved trauma are in their own individual psychotherapy concomitant with their participation in parent coaching.

Sometimes the parent's individual therapist has referred them for parent coaching and sometimes I recommend individual psychotherapy for the parent. For a few parents, their relationship with me was their first supportive relationship with a mental health professional and they did not feel comfortable seeking their own mental health services until midway through IoWA-PCIT treatment.

Given that we know there are effective interventions for unresolved attachment, it is obviously advantageous to have the parent involved in their own effective therapy while participating in parent coaching. It is also useful to be familiar with the type of intervention the parent is receiving so you can speak the same language as their individual therapist.

I find parents with unresolved attachment often benefit from mentalization-based therapy (Asen & Fonagy, 2011). Mentalization is a term that describes "seeing ourselves from the outside and seeing others from the inside" (Asen & Fonagy, 2011). The focus of mentalization-based therapy is helping patients improve their capacity to step into someone else's shoes and understand their experience, a capacity that is impaired in individuals who have unresolved attachment trauma. When I am coaching parents who are receiving mentalization-based therapy, I can make comments about what the child might be experiencing in order to help the parent better understand the child's experience.

Circle of Security (Powell et al., 2014) is another approach that fits well with IoWA-PCIT coaching and I have found to be especially helpful to parents with unresolved attachment. Parents who participate in the Circle of Security intervention (Powell et al., 2014) are able to identify the attachment experiences they failed to receive during their childhood and the experiences they would like to provide their children. During IoWA-PCIT coaching, I can reinforce the concepts the parent is learning in Circle of Security using language from the intervention. For example, when the child is engaged in exploration, I can talk about the child "going out on the circle" (Powell et al., 2014). During parent coaching, I also have opportunities to recognize the parent's grief for what they failed to receive and affirm their wish to provide a different experience for their child. For example, I might say, "I can see how you are helping her with her emotional regulation. I know that is something you wished your parents had helped you with as a child."

Another intervention that is useful in helping parents cope with unresolved trauma is exposure therapy. For parents who experienced abuse during their childhood, having them remember the trauma in a safe setting with a therapist can lead to resolution of their childhood abuse (Stovall-McClough & Cloitre, 2003). For parents with their own childhood abuse, exposure to their child acting in ways they acted as a child can be very upsetting. Controlled exposure to video clips that activate the parent's attachment system (e.g., a moment of positive parent–child interaction, a moment of separation, and a moment of reunion) and moments of challenging interactions can reduce mothers' negative attributions about their child (Schechter et al., 2006).

What the research on exposure therapy tells us is if we can keep anxiety from overwhelming the parent, exposure to reminders of loss or trauma in a safe setting can actually be healing. Our goal during IoWA-PCIT coaching is to keep the parent from becoming overwhelmed by anxiety—for both the sake of the parent and the sake of the child.

Prevalence of Unresolved Attachment

In community samples, 6–25% of adults exhibit unresolved attachment on the Adult Attachment Interview (AAI) (Bakermans-Kranenburg & van Ijzendoorn, 2009; Caspers et al., 2007). Among adults seeking treatment for borderline personality disorder, 32% exhibit unresolved attachment (Levy et al., 2006). Unresolved attachment is prevalent in parents of children with disorganized attachment (53%) (van Ijzendoorn, 1995) and parents participating in parent management training for a child with disruptive behavior (43%) (Routh et al., 1995).

Course of Treatment with Parents with Unresolved Attachment

The author of the article quoted earlier in this chapter, Gordon Marino (2015), attributes his ability to address his disorganizing childhood to his therapeutic relationship with Beatrice Beebe. I loved recognizing how Beatrice Beebe's insights from her research on attachment theory made it into their work together, work that, to Gordon Marino, was clearly different from his experience with other mental health professionals. He states, "It is almost as though we have forgotten the matchless healing power of relationships, a power that I can attest to, since I have been on the couch for almost 45 years with the same person" (Marino, 2015). It is a reminder that what it takes to heal from a disorganizing attachment relationship is a healing relationship.

I recognize that the length of time Beatrice Beebe and Gordon Marino spent working together may be discouraging to therapists thinking about helping parents with unresolved loss and trauma change their relationship with their child. I'm not suggesting that we will spend 45 years with parents with unresolved attachment. However, I think it is important that we be realistic about what it takes to create the type of long-term change we are working toward with families with unresolved attachment trauma. It is unfair to expect parents with unresolved attachment trauma, who often continue to live in disorganizing and traumatizing situations, to demonstrate the type of immediate response to IoWA-PCIT we see in secure dyads. When working with families with unresolved trauma, our first goal is establishing a safe, therapeutic relationship.

Our relationship with the parent and the parent's relationship with the child are two important allies against the ghosts that enter the playroom during IoWA-PCIT. Our goal is to use these relationships to help the parent stay grounded and in the moment with their child. We need to stay alert to the stressful conditions that may evoke intense and out-of-context affect in the parent. We need to be able to co-regulate the parent's affect so they can help the child co-regulate.

I spend more time in the playroom (instead of behind the mirror) when working with parents with unresolved attachment loss or trauma at the beginning of the session. I often spend a little time with the parent and me doing joint Child-Directed Interaction (CDI) with the child. Basically, both the parent and I are taking turns describing, reflecting, and praising the child. I describe this to parents as "team CDI"—a reminder of our partnership on behalf of their child.

Sometimes, despite my best efforts to keep the playroom a safe place for the parent and child, I find parents with unresolved attachment trauma becoming dysregulated. In these situations, my presence behind the mirror may not provide enough co-regulation for them to calm down. When a parent becomes dysregulated and seems unable to become more regulated with behind-the-mirror coaching, I sometimes go into the room and speak directly to the parent.

This happens most often during Parent-Directed Interaction (PDI), an especially stressful time for many dyads. When I notice a parent becoming more stressed—that is, displaying frightening or frightened behavior toward the child, I start out talking behind the mirror in a calm, soothing voice to the parent. I often remind them of things we had talked about during the PDI teach session. For example, saying that we had talked about how the hardest thing for them during PDI might be if their child called them names and telling them now that this is happening, and they are handling it. I note any ways of managing their anxiety that I might notice they themselves using, such as deep breathing, stretching, looking out the window, or coloring.

If the parent continues to appear frightening (e.g., yelling at the child) or frightened (e.g., cowering), I will enter the room. First, I talk directly to the parent. I acknowledge that this is a really difficult moment for them and their child and I am here to support them through it. I remind the parent of the ways they have learned to respond to their child in IoWA-PCIT. For example, if we are in PDI, I might remind the parent that their child is sitting in the time-out chair, and even though the child is yelling at them, they need to ignore the yelling and wait for the child to be quiet. I remind the parent that once their child is quiet, their child will have an opportunity to follow the command and get off the time-out chair. By reviewing these procedures with the parent, I am helping to keep them in the present, reminding them where they are and what happens next. This also provides a review for the child of what happens next. I stay in the room, providing coaching and reassurance for the parent through the PDI procedure. Once the child has completed the time-out procedure by following the command and the parent has returned to Child-Directed Interaction (CDI), I may join in the CDI—helping the child and parent become regulated by providing an extra dose of CDI.

Occasionally, when I see a parent becoming overwhelmed during interactions with their child, I will go into the playroom and offer the parent a break. This might occur during CDI or after a particularly challenging time-out procedure. I ask the parent if they would like to go get a drink of water or walk around for a minute. I reassure the child that the parent will be right back. Then I do CDI with the child while their parent takes a break. My goal is to communicate to the parent and child that sometimes parents need a break to take care of themselves and that is okay.

When working with parents with unresolved attachment, I schedule more parent-only sessions to continue holding the parent firmly in mind so they can keep the child in mind. Because it can be more difficult to repair ruptures in the relationship with parents with unresolved attachment, I can also address any ruptures in our relationship during these parent-only sessions.

During these parent-only sessions, I can ask the parent about their support system, ensure they felt supported by me during coaching, and address any times they felt unsupported by my coaching. For example, if the parent felt criticized or unsupported by my coaching, we can talk about it.

These sessions often start out focused on relatively minor (to me) ways in which the parent felt I did not support them—for example, my failure to remember which toys the parent did not want in the playroom. Although this lapse on my part may seem minor, I know that lack of recognition and support is often at the heart of unresolved attachment. If I want the parent to be able to provide a holding environment for their child, I need to be able to provide a holding environment for the parent.

So, I begin by respecting the parent's perspective that I failed to support them by forgetting which toys they did not want in the playroom. I find that acknowledging the ways I have let the parent down during the coaching often leads to a discussion of how the parent feels they were let down by their own parents and their deep desire not to let their child down in the same way. These discussions help me stay focused on the parent's intent for their child during coaching sessions.

The Bottom Line

When parents have unresolved attachment issues, we have an opportunity to provide a healing experience for both the parent and child. Specifically, our IoWA-PCIT coaching can provide the parent with an experience where they are supported through a stressful experience. A core component of working with parents with unresolved attachment is keeping their anxiety at a manageable level. In order to coach parents with unresolved attachment, it is useful to know about other interventions they have received to address their attachment anxiety. We also need to be explicit with the parent about how we can support them during the coaching, and we need to reinforce effective strategies for managing anxiety during our coaching. We need to hold the parent in mind during our coaching so the parent can hold the child in mind. Parents with their own attachment trauma have more difficulty trusting us and more difficulty repairing the relationship with us following ruptures. Parent-only sessions can be useful in building and maintaining our therapeutic alliance with parents with unresolved attachment.

References

Asen, E., & Fonagy, P. (2011). Mentalization-based therapeutic interventions for families. *Journal of Family Therapy, 34*, 1–24.
Bakermans-Kranenburg, M., & van Ijzendoorn, M. (2009). The first 10,000 adult attachment interviews: Distributions of adult attachment representations in clinical and non-clinical groups. *Attachment & Human Development, 11*(3), 223–263.
Caspers, K. M., Paradiso, S., Yucuis, R., Troutman, B., Arndt, S., & Philibert, R. (2009). Association between the serotonin transporter promoter polymorphism (5-HTTLPR) and adult unresolved attachment. *Developmental Psychology, 45*(1), 64–76.
Caspers, K. M., Yucuis, R., Troutman, B., Arndt, S., & Langbehn, D. (2007). A sibling adoption study of adult attachment: The influence of shared environment on attachment state of mind. *Attachment & Human Development, 9*(4), 375–391.
George, C., Kaplan, N., & Main, M. (1984). *Adult attachment interview*. University of California.
Levy, K., Meehan, K., Kelly, K., Reynoson, J., Weber, M., Clarkin, J., & Kernberg, O. (2006). Change in attachment patterns and reflective function in a randomized control trial of transference-focused pyschotherapy for borderline personality disorder. *Journal of Consulting and Clinical Psychology, 74*(6), 1027–1040.
Main, M. (2000). The organized categories of infant, child, and adult attachment: Flexible vs. inflexible attention under attachment-related stress. *Journal of the American Psychoanalytic Association, 48*, 1055–1096.
Marino, G. (2015). The long conversation. *The New York Times*. June 2.
Powell, B., Cooper, G., Hoffman, K., & Marvin, R. (2014). *The circle of security intervention: Enhancing attachment in early parent-child relationships*. The Guilford Press.
Putnam, F. (1992). Are alter personalities fragments or figments? *Psychoanalytic Inquiry, 12*, 95–111.
Routh, C., Hill, J., Steele, H., Elliott, C., & Dewey, M. (1995). Maternal attachment status, psychosocial stressors and problem behaviour: Follow-up after parent training courses for conduct disorder. *Journal of Child Psychology and Psychiatry, 36*(7), 1179–1198.
Schechter, D., Myers, M., Brunelli, S., Coates, S., Zeanah, C. H., Davies, M., … Liebowitz, M. (2006). Traumatized mothers can change their minds about their toddlers: Understanding how a novel use of videofeedback supports positive change of maternal attributions. *Infant Mental Health Journal, 27*(5), 429–447.
Stovall-McClough, K., & Cloitre, M. (2003). Reorganization of unresolved childhood traumatic memories following exposure therapy. *Annals of the New York Academy of Sciences, 1008*, 297–299.
van Ijzendoorn, M. (1995). Adult attachment representations, parental responsiveness, and infant attachment: A meta-analysis on the predictive validity of the adult attachment interview. *Psychological Bulletin, 117*(3), 387–403.

Chapter 15
Attachment Trauma: How to Tailor Coaching for Parents of Children in Foster Care

This chapter discusses how to use attachment-informed parent coaching to help children in foster care heal from the multiple layers of attachment trauma they have experienced. I describe how to help children in foster care develop healthier relationships with both foster and biological parents.

Challenges Faced by Young Children in Foster Care

As I mentioned in the preface to this book, babysitting young children in foster care was an experience that affected me deeply and led me to a long-term interest in addressing the emotional needs of young children. This work can be challenging. What keeps me going is the group of allies I have in this work. Over the course of my career, there have been significant advances in understanding and addressing the attachment trauma of young children in foster care.

In my chapter on disorganized attachment (Chap. 13), I noted that either loss or trauma can be associated with disorganized attachment. Young children in foster care have typically experienced both—maltreatment by a parent and loss of a parent.

Let me start by stating emphatically that, in general, placement in foster care is vastly superior to the alternative of placement in residential care. Early case studies by James and Joyce Robertson indicated that when a young child needed to be separated from their parent, placement in a foster home was vastly superior to placement in a residential treatment setting (Robertson & Robertson, 1989). These early observations by the Robertsons (1989) have been validated by a heartbreaking longitudinal study called the Bucharest Early Intervention Project (Nelson et al., 2014). The Bucharest Early Intervention Project was developed to look at how to reduce the problems faced by young children placed in institutional care in Romania, where large numbers of children were being reared in orphanages. In the Bucharest Early Intervention Project, young children either remained in the orphanage or were placed in a foster home. The children who were placed in foster care did better on a wide variety of social and emotional outcomes. These results are consistent with what we know about the importance of early relationships.

Foster children learn at an early age what we all must eventually face—the impermanence of our most important relationships. The child who is placed in foster care —either formally or informally—starts with the challenge of forming a new attachment relationship in the face of loss. Often, this loss was preceded by challenges in the attachment relationship that forced them to develop a particular strategy.

Attachment Myth That Damages Young Children in Foster Care

One of the challenges faced by foster parents and children in foster care is the prevalent myth among biological parents, foster parents themselves, and the professionals working with them (attorneys, guardian ad litems, social workers, and therapists) that children placed in out-of-home care should not become attached to their foster parents. I continue to hear therapists and social workers express concern when I mention improving the attachment relationship between foster parents and the young children in their care. One of the concerns I hear is that the child forming a strong attachment to their foster parent will make it too difficult for the child when they have to leave the foster home for reunification or placement in an adoptive home.

How does a foster parent respond to this? Do they do what will be most advantageous when the child returns to their home or finds a permanent placement, or do they provide the child with more nurturing? This is a question I struggled with a lot early in my career. Now I realize that it's not an either-or situation. I now clearly come down on the side of foster parents providing foster children with nurturing, just as I come down on the side of foster children needing to become attached to their foster parents. Just as the experience of having been neglected or maltreated is never entirely lost, the experience of having been cherished and cared for is never lost. In fact, experiencing positive caregiving from a foster parent actually contributes to more positive interactions with biological parents (Forte, 2015). Providing foster children with prompt, consistent, and appropriate responses to their attachment signals is a win-win situation.

I am surprised at the prevalence of this idea—that young children should not form a secure attachment to their foster parents—given the overwhelming data on the positive impact sensitively responsive foster parents can have on children coping with disruptions in their attachment relationships. It is not possible for young children to survive without becoming attached to an alternative parent. We have known since the early observational work of James and Joyce Robertson, conducted in the

1960s, that having an available, responsive caregiver lessens the profound emotional impact of being separated from a parent (Robertson & Robertson, 1989).

How Early Attachment Trauma Impacts Attachment Relationships

When thinking about the long-term impact of trauma and how to help children who have experienced early maltreatment by attachment figures, I have found Philip Bromberg's writings to be congruent with my way of thinking. In his book *The Shadow of the Tsunami and the Growth of the Relational Mind*, Bromberg (2011) describes how his adult psychoanalytic patients enact childhood traumatic experiences, ones they are unable to express verbally, as they interact with him. For example, Bromberg describes his interactions with a woman with unresolved attachment and dissociation resulting from a father who behaved sadistically toward her while simultaneously suggesting there must be something wrong with her for thinking someone as loving as him would ever want to hurt her. In other words, a perfect setup for disorganized/disoriented attachment. Bromberg (2011) describes an interaction where he realizes he is behaving toward her as her father had—pushing her to accept his reality of their relationship and behaving punitively toward her when she did not.

Just as psychoanalytic patients enact their attachment trauma with their psychoanalysts, foster children enact their attachment trauma with their foster parents. Our role as therapists is to help the child develop a secure and healthy attachment relationship with their foster parent, a relationship that will help sustain them during the separation from their parent and help them begin to internalize a secure working model of attachment. Although recollection of attachment trauma may occur, it is not the primary goal of our work. Our primary goal is helping the child develop healthier relationships with their parents (foster and biological).

The younger the child when the attachment trauma occurred, the more likely it is that the trauma will be part of who they are and how they see the world. What we would perceive as trauma (e.g., physical abuse or neglect by a parent) is just how the world is from their perspective. The processing of attachment trauma needs to be done in the context of a relationship, and the relationship where this is most likely to happen is in the relationship with the foster parent. But before the processing of trauma can begin, the foster parent needs to form a relationship with the child that is secure and healthy. The foster parent must provide the blueprint for this relationship as the child's blueprint is one that is based on previous attachment trauma.

Helping Young Children Heal from Attachment Trauma

When working with young children in foster care, there is sometimes the perception among therapists that if we aren't talking about the trauma, we aren't doing our job. Providing a place where children in foster care can talk about or play about their trauma is certainly an important part of healing—and the part of healing that I focused most on early in my career. What I have learned is that with early relational trauma, young children may not even realize it is trauma. When you grow up with attachment trauma, it is just how relationships are. Therefore, before young children can express their trauma, they need to be in a different type of relationship. We need to focus on providing them with an attachment relationship where they are seen, heard, and valued before they are able to express their trauma.

Providing young foster children with a relationship where their attachment signals are recognized and responded to is the first step, and perhaps the most important step, in helping them heal from attachment trauma. Through attachment-informed parent coaching, we are able to help foster parents provide this healing relationship.

As described above, young children in foster care often arrive with a number of their own attachment challenges. The first challenge they are facing is the loss of their attachment relationship with their biological parents. I'll never forget the 13-year-old patient who experienced the termination of her parents' rights due to neglect and abuse as her rights to having a relationship with them being terminated. Although this young woman had been referred to me with a diagnosis of "attachment disorder," I experienced something quite different in my interactions with her—a young woman who cared deeply about relationships and continued to grieve the loss of her biological family.

Of course, most children are unable to speak so eloquently about their loss. Instead, they respond in the way almost all infants and young children respond to disruptions in their attachment relationships. Some of the behaviors frequently seen in children separated from their parents are crying, being angry and defiant, and hitting or kicking (Gean et al., 1985; Robertson & Robertson, 1989). One of the tragedies for children caught up in the foster care system is that disruptions in attachment relationships beget disruptive behavior and disruptive behavior leads to more disruptions in attachment relationships. As children get older and have a longer history of disruptions in attachment relationships, they may present with a large array of problems associated with disorganized attachment including anxiety, depression, post-traumatic stress symptoms, and disruptive behavior.

Challenges Faced by Foster Parents

The types of emotional and behavioral problems seen in children in foster care are understandable given their experience with attachment figures. However, these behaviors are extremely challenging for foster families and place stress on the developing relationships. Foster parents often experience disruptive behaviors as rejecting. This makes it difficult for the foster parent to get close to the child and provide the nurturing the child so desperately needs.

Prior to being placed in foster care, children have typically experienced abuse or neglect that led to being removed from their home. Because of the circumstances that led to being removed, there is often an expectation on the part of foster parents and social workers that the child will be grateful for having been rescued from these difficult circumstances. Although this might make sense when viewed from the foster parents' perspective, when viewed from the child's perspective, it is easy to see why, instead of feeling grateful, the child can have difficulty trusting the new adults in their lives, given their history.

When coaching foster parents, I also try to keep in mind the challenging and difficult task of investing in and committing to a child who may not be with them long term. We know from research that how foster parents handle this uncertainty has enormous implications for their child's emotional development (Bernard & Dozier, 2011). For young children in foster care, the foster parent's commitment to them is even more important to the development of a secure attachment with the foster parent than the foster parent's sensitive responsiveness. One of the ways this commitment is communicated to the child is through the foster parent's delight in them (Bernard & Dozier, 2011). For children who have experienced attachment trauma, being appreciated and delighted in for who you are seems to be a powerful antidote to the devastating experiences of maltreatment.

Many of the foster parents I work with are exceptionally good parents. They pride themselves on their caregiving abilities and derive a great deal of satisfaction from parenting. Parenting a foster child who undermines their parenting self-efficacy is a blow to their confidence in their parenting ability. When I work with foster parents, it is typically because their current parenting strategies have not worked with the particular child referred to me for services.

Because young children tend to enact their previous attachment relationships with foster parents, their foster parents can find themselves pulled into behaving with these children in ways they could not previously have imagined. This can be a very unsettling experience. Foster parents have told me that their biological children have made statements like "You're so strict with her. You were never like that with us." The foster parent will say that they didn't have to be strict with their biological children because their biological children didn't exhibit the behavior problems they see in their foster children. Part of the task with foster parents is to provide them with a space where it is possible for them to reflect on how the characteristics of their foster child and their previous experiences contribute to the ways they are responding to the child. In addition to helping them reflect on the experience of being a foster parent, we provide opportunities to be coached in responding in different ways to their foster child and provide a relaxing and supportive space where they have the opportunity to enjoy time with their foster child.

While some foster parents can become overly strict and punitive when faced with a child who is angry and aggressive, other foster parents see past the behavior to the trauma that created it. Although it can be helpful for foster parents to be able to see how the child's aggression is associated with their previous attachment experiences, some of these foster parents may have difficulty setting limits with the child. With these foster parents, I talk about how being treated as a victim is not helpful for the child. If we excuse the child's aggression because we know it is the result of what happened to them, we are accepting the aggression that happened to them.

Child-Directed Interaction (CDI) with Foster Parents

Therapist-coached Child-Directed Interaction (CDI) gives foster parents the opportunity to see the child's behavior in a new light and to respond differently. It also provides an opportunity for the foster parent to express the delight in the child that we know is a critical component of healing from attachment trauma (Bernard & Dozier, 2011).

I have found that once the foster parent becomes adept at CDI, the foster child may begin expressing their trauma through play as a way to express and manage their feelings about their experiences—for example, having the mother doll hit the baby doll or leave the baby doll at home. Like therapists, foster parents tend to be helpers. In these moments of trauma play, foster parents sometimes want to fix the situation by telling the child not to hit the baby doll or not to leave the baby doll at home. When that happens, it is helpful for the therapist to hold a sacred space for the foster parent so they can hold it for the child. In other words, the therapist needs to acknowledge the distress evoked in the foster parent (and in the therapist) when witnessing the child's traumatic play. So, the therapist might say, for example, "This is really tough to see her hitting her baby doll. I suspect she may be telling us something about her experience with her parent."

The therapist needs to communicate that, as difficult as it is to observe the child's traumatic play, being a witness to the child's experience can provide another avenue of healing from her trauma. To convey this, the therapist might say, for example, "Your great play therapy allows her to work through her experiences through the play. This is so helpful for her to be able to share this with you." The therapist can model allowing the child to use play to express their trauma by providing the type of relationship they want the foster parent to provide the child. In other words, the therapist can allow the foster parent to have their feelings of distress *and* encourage the foster parent to accept the child using play to express their earlier traumas. For example, the therapist might say, "This is really important for her to be able to share her experiences with you through play." During these moments, I tell the foster parent how important it is to the child's healing that they provide the type of relationship that allows their child to heal. I might say, for example, "She is lucky to have you in her life. Your relationship will make a difference in her future."

Children may become embarrassed or ashamed about the play, recognizing at some level that they are revealing secrets about their family or themselves or reliving shame they felt during the original trauma. For example, I have seen children whisper when they begin to express their trauma through play. I have also seen children become angry and aggressive, identifying with an angry and aggressive parent. In this way, play therapy can become emotionally overwhelming for the child and foster parent.

When playing out the trauma becomes dysregulating for the child, "regular CDI" (i.e., CDI that is not focused on trauma) can help the child and foster parent become regulated again. Regular CDI is an experiential reminder of a different type of attachment relationship—one where the child is seen (behavior descriptions), heard (reflections), and valued (labeled praise). Part of our role as therapists is to guide the parent in helping the child use play to express traumatic experiences without becoming overwhelmed by the traumatic play. Working to help the foster parent titrate the child's exposure to traumatic memories in a way that allows the child and the foster parent to feel safe is a difficult balancing act. I find the structure of CDI very helpful in this regard because the child cannot engage in dangerous and destructive behavior during CDI. This means that the child, the foster parent, and the therapist all know that if the play escalates into real-life dangerous or destructive behavior, special play ends. Some therapists are concerned that ending special play for a traumatized child who has become destructive or aggressive invalidates the child's experience of sharing their trauma narrative. I believe the opposite is true—it is consistent with our message that destructive and aggressive behavior in relationships is not acceptable. Our goal is to teach children a new way of being in relationships—one where it is safe to talk or play about anything, but it is not acceptable to be harmful to themselves or others.

It's important to remember that we don't have to let the dysregulation escalate to the point where the play needs to end. Our goal, in trying to achieve a balance between safety and expressing trauma, is to look for clues that the child is becoming overwhelmed. If we notice the child's play is becoming increasingly out of control, we can coach the foster parent to begin playing separately from the child—and describing what they are doing. The foster parent then has the opportunity to reinforce the child's ability to calm down and regroup after an emotionally upsetting experience.

Parent-Directed Interaction (PDI) with Foster Parents

It is important to teach foster parents how to set limits safely and effectively with young children who have been maltreated and experienced attachment disruptions. This phase of IoWA-PCIT can be especially troubling for therapists and foster parents due to concerns about retraumatizing the child. It is useful to have as many details as possible about the maltreatment that led to the child being placed in foster care so we can take this into account when we move to PDI. For example, if the child has experienced physical and/or verbal abuse for misbehaving, the PDI procedure may evoke traumatic memories about what happened in the past when they misbehaved. Or, if the child has been neglected and left alone for periods of time, sending them to their room for getting off the time-out chair may evoke traumatic memories of being left alone.

My experience of coaching foster parents in PDI did not reflect the above concerns about the potential negative impact of PDI on young children in foster care. Initially, I too had concerns about coaching PDI with children in foster care. However, it was often necessary to help foster parents set limits due to the child's level of disruptive behavior and aggression, problems that decreased but did not go away in CDI.

The majority of the time, I have followed the standard PDI protocol, as laid out in the chapter on setting limits (Chap. 5). In other words, noncompliance with a command results in a warning, followed by time-out in a chair, followed by being sent to their room if they are unable to take time-out in a chair. However, I am sensitive to the child's previous maltreatment history, and if necessary, I make adaptations to the protocol. So, for example, I ensure foster parents do 5–10 minutes of CDI before giving a command. In this way, I set the child up for success—providing them with an extra dose of attachment priming (Over & Carpenter, 2009; Stupica et al., 2019) before they're expected to follow a command.

For children whose maltreatment history includes being left alone, I often modify the procedure, so they are not left in a room alone as a consequence of getting off the time-out chair. In my consultation with foster parents, we discuss the standard procedure and modifications that make sense given their child's level of behavior problems and maltreatment history. One strategy I have used, based on the concept of errorless compliance training (Rames-LaPointe et al., 2014), is to ignore noncompliance when PDI is first introduced (instead of using time-out for noncompliance). This provides an opportunity for the child to get experience with following directions in a low-stress situation—one where their compliance is praised and there is no consequence of noncompliance. This slow rollout of PDI also allows the foster parent to see their child following directions in an environment where noncompliance and negative consequences for noncompliance aren't an issue, a powerful reminder of the importance of their praise and relationship to the child. This also provides me with information about the possible pacing of commands in subsequent sessions, so we can slowly introduce time-out for noncompliance. Another modification I have used is for the child to lose a privilege for getting off the time-out chair, as detailed in the UC Davis PCIT for Traumatized Children protocol available at https://pcit.ucdavis.edu/forms/pdi-forms/.

I find that young children in foster care appreciate the predictability of the PDI procedure. They find it reassuring to know exactly what will happen if they do not follow the parent's commands—and what will happen if they do. Rather than being retraumatizing, I find that PDI can be healing for young children in foster care. They are able to have a different experience with a parent, an experience where having a parent set limits is regulating and reassuring rather than dysregulating.

Working with Biological Parents of Young Children in Foster Care

Whenever possible, I try to coach the biological parent of the foster child in IoWA-PCIT. Ideally, these sessions are on a different day or time than the appointments with the foster parent, but the foster parent transports the child to the session. I feel strongly that as long as the biological parents continue to be involved in their child's life, they should have the opportunity to improve their relationship with their child. Again, this is based on my understanding of the power of attachment relationships—even, or perhaps especially, when those relationships have been harmful to the child. I want to be able to provide support for biological parents to repair their relationship with their child to the extent possible—even if they never live with their child again and even if their parental rights are eventually terminated.

Working with biological parents who have maltreated their children is tough work. When I read the reports of what has happened and the ways in which the biological parent has endangered their child, I feel angry. When I get to know the biological parents of children in foster care, I often come to understand the challenges and wounds that have led them to inflict such pain on their child.

I have found that many biological parents whose children are in foster care are very receptive to being involved in IoWA-PCIT. The biological parents of young children in foster care often seem to have every card stacked against them—their own history of attachment trauma, their own mental health issues, poverty, and a social services system that often feels like the enemy to them. I am inspired by the biological parents who have been able to overcome these hurdles and provide their children with the type of positive parenting they did not receive during their childhood.

There is a tendency to continue to blame biological parents for the child's problems after the child is placed in foster care. While this is understandable given the circumstances leading to placement in foster care, the biological parent cannot go back in time and undo the damage they have done in their relationship with their child. Learning new skills to address the child's problems shifts the focus to using these new skills, improving the biological parent's relationship with the child, and promoting healthy child development. The same is true for foster parents. One of the advantages of teaching both the foster and the biological parent to use CDI skills with the child is that there is a shared set of principles for healthy parenting.

When Attachment-Informed Parent Coaching with Biological Parents of Children in Foster Care Is Not Appropriate

There are situations where attachment-informed parent coaching should not be done with biological parents. Despite my commitment to improving the child–parent relationship, there are situations where dyadic work is not appropriate and other interventions need to be implemented. One of these situations is parents who have sexually abused their child. In cases where a parent has sexually abused a child, I do not coach the sexual abuse perpetrator in CDI or PDI. In these cases, Trauma-Focused Cognitive Behavioral Therapy (TF-CBT) (Cohen & Mannarino, 1996, 1997) is a good therapeutic option. TF-CBT provides psychoeducation about the impact of trauma and teaches the child relaxation and affective modulation skills. In TF-CBT, the therapist works directly with the child on developing a trauma narrative that is shared with parents when appropriate.

There are also times when physical abuse or neglect by the biological parent has been so severe that exposing the child to interactions with the parent is too overwhelming for the child. In these situations, I meet with the parent for parent-only sessions, and we work on activities that can be used to provide the child gradual exposure to the parent in a safe situation. For example, I may start with helping the parent write cards and letters to the child and work up to the parent making brief videos for the child. I then gradually share these cards, letters, and videos during individual sessions with the child or CDI sessions with the child and the foster parent, carefully titrating the exposure to keep the child from becoming overwhelmed. In these situations, I also teach the biological parent the PRIDE skills (i.e., **P**raise, **R**eflect, **I**mitate, **D**escribe, and **E**njoy). In my clinical experience, the biological parents of children in foster care are often parenting other children who are still in the home. My hope is to provide these parents with parenting tools and new models for positive interaction with all their children.

Another situation where I wait to coach the biological parent is when the parent has ongoing issues with severe mental illness and/or substance abuse that prevent them from acknowledging the pain they have caused their child or committing to making changes in their interactions. It is still useful for the IoWA-PCIT therapist to have parent-only sessions with the parent in this situation. These sessions acknowledge the parent's ongoing role in the child's life and the therapist's commitment to improving the relationship between parent and child.

Working with Older Children and Adolescents in Foster Care

Older children and adolescents in the foster care system tend to have even larger wounds than young children. These relationships can be even more challenging due to the layers of attachment trauma and lack of consistent relationships in the child's life. But, like young children in foster care, older children continue to care deeply about relationships and want to be seen, heard, and valued by adults. The principles described in this chapter can be adapted to older children and adolescents in foster care. Praising, reflecting, and, most importantly, enjoying time with older children and adolescents can provide them with the experience of a different kind of relationship and set the stage for them to be a different kind of parent when they have children.

Despite the challenges faced by older children and adolescents in foster care, research indicates it is never too late for these children and young people to develop a secure attachment with their foster parents (Joseph et al., 2014). In one study, almost half of the adolescents in foster care had a secure attachment with their foster mother and foster father (Joseph et al., 2014). Furthermore, adolescents with more secure relationships with their foster parents had fewer symptoms of disruptive behavior.

The Bottom Line

Children in foster care need parents who are sensitively responsive to their attachment cues, to heal from attachment trauma. They also need parents who set limits on their behavior. In other words, children in foster care need what every child needs. Meeting the attachment needs of children in foster care can be especially challenging. The attachment trauma and disruptions they have experienced contribute to their engaging in behaviors that interfere with the parent's ability to meet their attachment needs. Our parent coaching can help foster parents respond sensitively to the child's attachment needs, provide sensitive discipline, and help the child begin healing from attachment trauma. It can also help biological parents begin to repair their relationships with their children.

References

Bernard, K., & Dozier, M. (2011). This is my baby: Foster parents' feelings of commitment and displays of delight. *Infant Mental Health Journal, 32*(2), 251–262.

Bromberg, P. (2011). *The shadow of the tsunami and the growth of the relational mind.* Taylor & Francis Group, LLC.

Cohen, J., & Mannarino, A. (1996). A treatment outcome study for sexually abused preschool children: Initial findings. *Journal of the American Academy of Child and Adolescent Psychiatry, 35,* 42–50.

Cohen, J., & Mannarino, A. (1997). A treatment study for sexually abused preschool children: Outcome during a one year follow-up. *Journal of the American Academy of Child and Adolescent Psychiatry, 36,* 1228–1235.

Forte, L. (2015). *When should we intervene? PCIT for foster children in reunification.* University of California Davis.

Gean, M., Gillmore, J., & Dowler, J. (1985). Infants and toddlers in supervised custody: A pilot study for visitation. *Journal of the American Academy of Child and Adolescent Psychiatry, 24*(5), 608–612.

Joseph, M., O'Connor, T., Briskman, J., Maughn, B., & Scott, S. (2014). The formation of secure new attachments by children who were maltreated: An observational study of adolescents in foster care. *Development and Psychopathology, 26*(1), 67–80.

Nelson, C., Fox, N., & Zeanah, C. H. (2014). *Romania's abandoned children: Deprivation, brain development, and the struggle for recovery.* Harvard University Press.

Over, H., & Carpenter, M. (2009). Attachment priming improves prosocial behavior in 18-month-olds. *Psychological Science, 20*(10), 1189–1193.

Rames-LaPointe, J., Hixson, M., Niec, L., & Rhymer, K. (2014). Evaluation of errorless compliance training in a general education classroom. *Behavioral Interventions, 29*(3), 253–267.

Robertson, J., & Robertson, J. (1989). *Separation and the very young*. Free Association Books.

Stupica, B., Brett, B., Woodhouse, S. S., & Cassidy, J. (2019). Attachment security priming decreases Children's physiological response to threat. *Child Development, 90*(4), 1254–1271.

Chapter 16
Adoption and Attachment: How to Tailor Coaching for Parents of Adopted Children

This chapter discusses how to tailor parent coaching when working with adopted children and their parents. This chapter describes some of the unique challenges faced by adopted children and their parents and how to use psychoeducation about the development of secure attachment in work with adopted children and their parents.

In Mary Ainsworth's first book, *Infancy in Uganda,* she provides a vivid description of a family who asked her to adopt their child, Paulo (Ainsworth, 1967). Ainsworth describes Paulo's family as relatively affluent and describes the biological child–mother attachment relationship as secure. According to Ainsworth, Paulo's parents determined that Ainsworth could provide their child with opportunities in Canada that they were unable to provide in Uganda. They also noted that Ainsworth "clearly loved him and would be good to him" (Ainsworth, 1967). Ainsworth did not adopt Paulo. But Paulo's father wrote Ainsworth annual letters long after the research was completed, updating her on Paulo and the rest of the family.

My reason for sharing this story from Ainsworth's (1967) research is to point out the complexity of the relationship between attachment and adoption. Each adoption story is unique. If Paulo had been adopted by Ainsworth, his story would have been considerably different from that of another older child who was, for example, adopted following placement in foster care.

I have helped adoptive parents think through what they want to say to their child about why the child isn't able to live with their biological parents. My guidance for thinking about these discussions comes from my understanding of how securely attached dyads communicate. That is, the communication should be clear and direct. Children should be comfortable asking questions so that adoptive parents will be able to answer them. General openness to discussing the adoption story is at least as important as the specifics of the story.

Attachment and Adoption

Because of the unique circumstances associated with adoption, there is a great deal of interest in attachment in adoptive families. Many therapists and adoptive families are surprised to learn that adoption per se is not associated with insecure attachment. The rate of secure attachment in children adopted before 12 months of age is the same as the rate in nonadopted children (van den Dries et al., 2009). In a unique study of families that included both adopted and biological children, my colleagues and I examined the working model of attachment of siblings who were not biologically related (Caspers et al., 2007). Secure attachment was the norm for both the adopted and biological children. Furthermore, the concordance between the siblings' attachment was high (Caspers et al., 2007). In other words, if the biological child had a secure working model of attachment, the adopted child was highly likely to have a secure working model of attachment as well.

Working with Adopted Children and Their Parents

Parents of adopted children are often especially concerned about the nature of their attachment relationship with their child. They don't take it for granted that their child will have a positive, secure attachment relationship with them. I also find that parents of adopted children are more likely to attribute their child's behavior problems to problems in the attachment relationship.

Many of the adoptive parents who seek treatment for their child's behavioral or emotional problems are concerned that their child has reactive attachment disorder. However, when I conduct an evaluation, I almost always find the child is clearly attached to the parent and often has a secure attachment (Troutman, 2016). Understanding and resolving this discrepancy is an important piece of my work with adoptive families.

Part of the discrepancy seems to be due to adoptive parents' expectations regarding attachment. Consequently, I find it important to have adoptive parents describe what they think a secure child–parent attachment relationship looks like. Often, the relationship they describe is not a realistic portrayal of the typical secure child–parent relationship. For this reason, I find psychoeducation about the development of attachment to be especially helpful in working with parents of adopted children. My psychoeducation with adoptive parents often focuses on educating them about the attachment/exploration balance in secure attachment, and the evidence for this balance in their relationship with their child.

The preschool Strange Situation Procedure I conduct as part of an initial attachment-informed assessment (described in Chap. 3) is especially useful in working with parents of adopted children. I have found the video review of the Strange Situation Procedure to be helpful in working with parents of adopted children. I schedule a session without the child present where the parent and I can view the parent's interaction with the child during the Strange Situation Procedure. As we watch this together, I am able to point out the indicators of healthy attachment I see during the taped interaction. I am also able to discuss the parents' perceptions of the interaction and address their concerns. This often reassures parents of adopted children that their child is securely attached to them.

During Child-Directed Interaction (CDI) coaching, I have additional opportunities to make observations about the attachment relationship between the child and parent. I am able to expand the parent's view of healthy attachment to include both the ways in which they scaffold their child's exploration and the ways in which the child seeks comfort when distressed.

In working with parents of adopted children, it is useful to make a distinction between children adopted as infants and children adopted at an older age following loss and/or trauma. For children adopted as infants, being adopted is less likely to be a factor in the nature of their attachment relationship with their parents. As noted earlier, children adopted as infants are just as likely to have a secure attachment relationship with their parents as biological children (Caspers et al., 2007; van den Dries et al., 2009). Also, because the attachment relationship is developed during the first year of life, the quality of the attachment relationship is likely to be the result of the experiences with their adoptive parent, and their adoptive parents' working model of attachment, rather than previous attachment experiences.

When working with children who were adopted when they were older, we are also addressing the attachment trauma associated with their early experiences. As described in the previous chapter on children in foster care (Chap. 15), the primary focus of the work with adopted children is on building a more positive relationship with their adoptive parents. This relationship becomes the secure base from which the child can eventually explore their previous traumatic attachment experiences. As noted in Chap. 15, children tend to bring their previous strategies or patterns of attachment into their new relationships, along with the wounds from these relationships.

For adoptive parents with a secure working model of attachment, overcoming these previous strategies is easier than for adoptive parents who have dismissing, preoccupied, or unresolved working models. Adoptive parents with secure working models of attachment seem to be able to look past the child's strategy—for example, pushing the parent away—and see the attachment need underneath the strategy. Thus, children with maltreatment histories who are adopted by a parent with secure attachment are likely to develop a secure attachment relationship with their adoptive parents despite their early history (Steele et al., 2008). When working with adoptive parents who don't have a secure attachment, we need to tailor our coaching to the parent's insecure working model, as described in Chaps. 10, 12, and 14.

When working with older children who have been adopted following maltreatment, I find it useful to do a timeline of the child's placements at the initial evaluation. That is, I try to gather information about the child's attachment history prior to placement in the adoptive home. This timeline can be useful in understanding the child's seemingly inexplicable reactions to certain situations. For example, it can uncover why the child reacts to indicators of seasonal changes such as Halloween decorations or changes in the weather, which may be reminders of previous losses or trauma. This attachment history helps me be sensitive to the child's perception. It gives me a sense of the length of time it may take before the child begins to trust that their relationship with their adoptive parents will be stable and secure. From the perspective of a child, attachment to a parent is a process that is distinct and separate from the legal decisions regarding who their parent is. CDI can facilitate the attachment process by providing a time where the child feels seen, heard, and appreciated by the parent. A small study of adopted children with disruptive behavior showed that IoWA-PCIT was extremely effective in reducing disruptive behavior (Troutman, 2016).

"Forever home" is a phrase frequently used by social workers and others to explain adoption to children adopted from the foster care system. I believe the use of this language reflects our heartfelt wish that the child has found a permanent home, one that provides the care they deserve. Unfortunately, it does not reflect the child's reality. Having a forever home is not congruent with the child's experience and telling them their new home is permanent does not make it so. As noted in Chap. 15, children adopted from the foster care system know well the impermanence of attachment relationships. It is important to be sensitive to the child's experience, giving them the opportunity to build trust over time through consistent and predictable interactions with their adoptive parents.

As with foster children (Chap. 15), Parent-Directed Interaction (PDI) is also an important component of work with children who have been adopted. PDI provides the child with the experience of predictable, consistent limits. It also allows the child to experience the normal rupture and repair that is a part of healthy relationships. That is, in PDI they learn that ruptures or conflicts in relationships can be followed by repair.

The Bottom Line

Attachment seems to have a special meaning in adoptive families. When working with adoptive families, it is important to recognize the unique questions and concerns of adoptive families in a manner that is grounded in research. In children adopted as infants, rates of secure attachment are comparable to rates in nonadopted children. Children who are adopted following loss and trauma have greater struggles with developing a secure attachment relationship with their adoptive parents. However, the building blocks for overcoming these obstacles and developing a secure attachment are the same as in other families—a sensitively responsive parent, a relationship where the child is seen, heard, and appreciated, and a relationship that provides appropriate limits. Attachment-informed parent coaching can recognize and reinforce the developing attachment relationship, providing a secure base for addressing previous attachment trauma.

References

Ainsworth, M. (1967). *Infancy in Uganda*. Johns Hopkins Press.

Caspers, K. M., Yucuis, R., Troutman, B., Arndt, S., & Langbehn, D. (2007). A sibling adoption study of adult attachment: The influence of shared environment on attachment state of mind. *Attachment & Human Development, 9*(4), 375–391.

Steele, M., Hodges, J., Kaniuk, J., Steele, H., Hillman, S., & Asquith, K. (2008). Forecasting outcomes in previously maltreated children: The use of the AAI in a longitudinal adoption study. In H. Steele & M. Steele (Eds.), *Clinical applications of the adult attachment interview*. The Guilford Press.

Troutman, B. (2016). Integrated behaviorism and attachment theory approach to reducing disruptive behavior in young adoptees. In K. Alvarez (Ed.), *Parent-child interactions and relationships: Perceptions, practices, and developmental outcomes* (pp. 61–74). Nova Publishers.

van den Dries, L., Juffer, F., van Ijzendoorn, M., & Bakermans-Kranenburg, M. (2009). Fostering security? A meta-analysis of attachment in adopted children. *Children and Youth Services Review, 31*(3), 410–421.

Chapter 17
Behind the Mirror: Learning and Growing as an Attachment-Informed Therapist

In this chapter, I describe how the experience of coaching parents of young children changes us and provides us with a unique opportunity to learn about our own working model of attachment. I discuss how the therapist's working model of attachment is communicated to their patients. I also discuss the lessons I've learned from coaching parents who have different working models of attachment than mine.

Growing as an Attachment-Informed Therapist

The person I am now is not the same person I was in my twenties when I first coached parents from behind a one-way mirror. Being genuine and authentic is a critical component in developing a therapeutic relationship with parents and children. Growing as an attachment-informed therapist means embracing who we are and reflecting on what we bring to the therapeutic relationships we form with the parents and children we work with.

The role of the therapist's self-disclosure in psychotherapy is one that has evolved over time. As more relationship-focused approaches to psychotherapy have become prominent, there has been more emphasis on the therapist's self-disclosure regarding their experience of the patient (Bromberg, 1998). I find that self-disclosure is especially relevant in an attachment-informed approach to parent coaching as there is the potential when coaching from behind a one-way mirror for the therapist to come across as judgmental or critical.

Using an attachment-informed approach when working with young children and their parents provides us with a unique, and not always welcome, opportunity to expand our understanding of our own working models of attachment. We may be behind a one-way mirror while coaching parents, but we can't hide who we are—from the parents we're coaching or from ourselves. We are changed by each family we work with, having new experiences and learning new things about ourselves.

There is something unique about the relationship formed when you are coaching in the moment while parents interact with their child. The parents we work with learn about us in ways we could not anticipate—and reflect ourselves back to us in ways we cannot anticipate.

I have had the opportunity to experience these growing pains myself as well as to see them in the therapists who attend my workshops. The first glimpse into our own working models can be like a kick in the gut—a recognition that our way of viewing the world and relationships may be limiting us in ways we weren't even aware of. As with the parents we work with, it is painful to recognize this truth. But it is also freeing. Recognizing that our road map for how to get our attachment needs met may not always take us where we want to go can help us explore new ways of being in relationships.

How Therapists' Working Models of Attachment Impact Their Communication with Patients

Just as a patient's working model of attachment impacts how they communicate with their therapist (Miller-Bottome et al., 2017, 2019; Talia et al., 2014; 2015), a therapist's working model of attachment impacts how the therapist communicates with their patients (Talia et al., 2020). Talia et al. (2020) developed the Therapist Attunement Scales (TASc), a method for coding therapy transcripts, in order to better understand how the therapist's working model of attachment impacted the therapist's communication with their patient during a therapy session. In a study of 50 psychodynamic therapists in Italy, the therapist's working model of attachment, as assessed by the Adult Attachment Interview (AAI), correlated with how they communicated with their patient during a psychotherapy session (Talia et al., 2020). I find this research helpful in thinking about how our own working model of attachment influences our communication with our patients. Understanding our own working model can help us understand where we may have difficulty supporting families and where we may be especially helpful. Interestingly, we may be most helpful to parents whose working model is slightly different than ours (Dozier et al., 1994). If you're someone who is very comfortable with supporting exploration but not so comfortable with supporting attachment (i.e., a bit more dismissing), you may be especially helpful when coaching parents who struggle with supporting exploration (i.e., parents who are a bit more preoccupied).

When reading the following descriptions of how therapists with different working models of attachment communicate with their patients, it is possible you may find you have communicated in ways that are associated with insecure working models. If so, you're not alone. When watching videos of my parent coaching, I see some truly cringeworthy moments where I said things to parents and children that were less than secure and therapeutic—the coaching moments that I left out of this book.

I have come to believe that showing who we really are to the families we work with is important, and perhaps inevitable. My goal is not that you learn to "sound like" a secure therapist but that you have a greater understanding of your working model and what your patients probably already know about the attachment lens you bring to parent coaching.

What Secure Therapists Sound Like When Communicating with Their Patients

There is no evidence that secure attachment is more or less common in psychotherapists than in the general population, with 62% of psychotherapists coded as secure on the Adult Attachment Interview (AAI) in a sample of Italian psychodynamic psychotherapists (Talia et al., 2020). Talia et al.'s research (2018) finds that secure psychotherapists ask questions or state ideas in a way that allows the patient to agree or disagree with them—allowing the patient to use them as a secure base to explore new ideas. Therapists with a secure working model of attachment communicate with their patients in ways that provide empathic validation for their patient's experience and suggest reasons the patient might be having a particular feeling. Secure therapists are more likely to communicate with their patients in ways that facilitate rapport and enhance the therapeutic alliance. Therapists with a secure working model of attachment share their positive feelings toward the patient, the patient's progress in psychotherapy, or something positive the patient said or did.

In my experience, secure therapists are willing to be vulnerable enough to admit they don't always have the answers. When coaching parents, they are willing to say things like "Whoa—what do you think about him standing on a chair? Is that dangerous?" They are also willing to admit mistakes and apologize, saying things like "Sorry about forgetting to have his favorite dinosaurs in there today." Or, "That was not a great command I had you give him. Sorry about that."

When coaching parents, I find it helpful to think about stepping in and out of the parent's perceptions. Secure therapists are able to step into the parent's working model and see the child from the parent's perspective and then step out of the parent's working model and offer their own perspective, saying things like "I saw you wince. It looks like you thought he might hit you with that plane when he flew it near your head." (This is an example of stepping in.) "I wonder if he got excited about flying his plane and didn't realize he might scare you." (This is an example of stepping out.)

All IoWA-PCIT therapists praise parents and children. Giving meaningful, heartfelt praise seems to come easier for secure therapists who already approach life with gratitude. I believe the focus on noticing and acknowledging positive interactions in IoWA-PCIT coaching helps us become more secure as we ourselves become more adept at noticing and valuing the ordinary magic in our own lives as well as in the lives of the families we coach.

Our own working models of attachment are especially likely to become activated when we're under stress. Stressful moments can often occur during parent coaching sessions—for example, when a child engages in dangerous or destructive behavior during a Child-Directed Interaction (CDI) session. For most therapists, initial Parent-Directed Interaction (PDI) sessions are among the most stressful. The distress of a young child in the time-out chair often evokes our own working models and ways of coping with distress. Therapists with secure working models of attachment check in with the parent to see how they are doing in these stressful moments—for example, "It seems like he is having a hard time on the time-out chair. How are you doing?"

What Dismissing Therapists Sound Like When Communicating with Their Patients

In the study of Italian psychotherapists described earlier, 22% had a dismissing working model of attachment on the AAI (Talia et al., 2020). Talia et al.'s (2020) research finds that dismissing therapists tend to downplay or normalize their patient's distress, just as dismissing parents downplay their child's distress. For example, dismissing therapists are more likely to respond to expressions of patient distress by suggesting the patient is a little upset or a bit angry (rather than suggesting they're very upset or angry, or just saying they seem upset or angry). Therapists with a dismissing working model of attachment also tend to normalize the patient's feelings by tying them to external events and suggesting the patient's feelings are common or typical. For a dismissing therapist, telling a patient their feelings are normal sounds reassuring because it would be reassuring for them. But it can be a way of detaching from their patient's feelings rather than attuning to the feelings.

Many of the problems that parents seek help with from therapists *are* a normal part of development. But since dismissing therapists tend to downplay distress, their attempts to reassure a parent by telling them that their child's disruptive behavior is normal or age-appropriate can come across as insensitive and fail to validate a parent's concerns. By detaching from the parent's concerns and not validating the parent's feelings about their child, their normalization of the child's difficulties can seem harsh and critical.

In my experience, dismissing therapists also tend to downplay the child's distress when coaching parents, saying things like "He's just crying to get your attention." Or, "He seems to be overreacting to his tower falling over." Attachment-informed parent coaching may be especially challenging for therapists with a dismissing state of mind (Dozier & Bernard, 2019). When faced with an infant's or young child's distress and a dismissing parent, they tend to revert to long-held beliefs that responding to a child's distress may spoil the child.

Dismissing therapists have a hard time stepping into the parent or child's working model, struggling to understand their perceptions or struggles. Although they are excellent at stepping out of the parent and child's working models and offering alternative perspectives and actions, dismissing therapists seem more likely to report that parents are resistant to their recommendations or coaching since they have not stepped in and seen the situation from the parent's and child's perspective. During stressful moments, dismissing therapists tend to ignore or downplay the parent's and child's distress, saying things like "Just follow the protocol and ignore his crying on the time-out chair." Or, "He is learning you won't give in just because he is upset."

What Preoccupied Therapists Sound Like When Communicating with Their Patients

In the study of psychodynamic Italian therapists described earlier, 12% were classified as preoccupied on the AAI (Talia et al., 2020). Therapists with a preoccupied working model of attachment use ways of communicating that have been labeled as coercive in Talia and colleagues' research (Talia et al., 2020). Just as patients with preoccupied working models of attachment communicate in ways that don't allow the therapist to have their own opinion, preoccupied therapists communicate in ways that don't allow the patient to have their own opinion. Preoccupied therapists are so focused on wanting to be on the same page with the patient that they don't allow the patient to explore issues for themselves. For example, the patient brings up a conflict with a family member and the preoccupied therapist states with certainty—"Your family member is angry because you are trying to express your own opinion." The therapist doesn't check in with the patient to see if this is how the patient experienced the conflict, closing off the possibility of exploration.

In my experience, therapists with a preoccupied working model can become so focused on their relationship with the parent that they forget about the needs of the child. For example, preoccupied therapists may be so focused on the parent's distress about the child's behavior that they begin to describe the child's behavior in a way that does not allow the parent to explore new ways of perceiving the child. The preoccupied therapist may interpret the child's behavior as doing things just to get under the parent's skin and may say things like "He's just doing that to annoy you." They don't offer alternative explanations for the behavior that might allow the parent to begin exploring other possible reasons for the child's behavior. Preoccupied therapists are adept at stepping into the parent's state of mind and seeing the problem from the parent's point of view. However, they struggle with stepping out and offering the parent alternative perspectives. In stressful moments, preoccupied therapists tell the parent how to feel rather than asking how they're feeling, saying things like "It must be traumatic for you to listen to him crying."

Disorganizing Moments in Parent Coaching

All therapists have experienced losses and traumas. Working with young children and their parents has a way of poking us in these sore spots. Our own unresolved losses and traumas, especially those associated with early-childhood experiences, can be triggered during parent coaching. Although this is true for all psychotherapy, I think parent coaching can be especially triggering. We are not just discussing early-childhood experiences, we are living these experiences with the child, when, for example, we see a parent criticize the child for not picking up toys fast enough or not knowing how to tie their shoe. Paying attention to our own visceral responses to the dyads we're coaching can help us recognize when we may be reacting based on our own childhood experiences.

When the therapist's previous loss or trauma is too similar to that of the parent or child and the therapist has too many unresolved sore spots, parent coaching can be retraumatizing for the therapist. In these situations, therapists can feel overpowered by strong, intense feelings about the parent and child that affect the therapist's perceptions of the situation—for example, experiencing an aggressive 2-year-old as dangerous, experiencing a 3-year-old who calls his mother a poopy-head as verbally aggressive, or experiencing a parent who criticizes his child for picking up toys slowly as abusive. For therapists with unresolved loss or trauma, stressful moments can result in the therapist feeling as though they themselves are experiencing the distress rather than coaching the parent through their child's distress.

When a therapist is experiencing strong, intense feelings about a family they're coaching that leads them to stray from the IoWA-PCIT model, I recommend discussing this with a trusted colleague or supervisor (reflective supervision) or with their own therapist. Just as parents will face difficult issues from their past for the sake of their children, therapists can be motivated to face difficult issues from their past for the sake of the families they coach.

What I've Learned from Coaching Parents with Different Working Models of Attachment

Coaching children and parents with different working models of attachment from our own is like visiting a different culture—we wonder what it would be like to live there and it makes us reflect on our own culture. I'm fascinated by how I am different with each family I coach. I find myself talking in ways that are more like the family's culture than my own, almost like picking up the local accent when visiting another country. Below are some of the lessons I've learned from the different working models I have been privileged to visit.

What I've Learned from Working with Secure Dyads

It is hard to visit secure dyads without wanting to live there. Maybe I don't exactly want to be part of their family but it sure is fun to visit. I love the ease with which they communicate with each other—including voicing negative feelings and being comfortable with conflict. Of course, I also love the way their affection and positive comments extend to me and the gratitude they express for our work together. And, when we arrive at the graduation session that marks the end of treatment, I'm sad that I will no longer be included in their family. Secure dyads have taught me to appreciate the diversity of ways to be in relationship and have modeled flexibility with how they make our work together a part of their unique family culture.

What I've Learned from Working with Avoidant Dyads

Visiting avoidant dyads is like running a marathon or climbing a mountain for your vacation trip—exhausting and focused on achievement. Working with dismissing parents has taught me to accept and understand my need to do things on my own and to avoid asking for help. As with the physical landscapes of our childhoods, there is an appreciation for this landscape that cannot be matched by other, more distant lands. I admire the grit of avoidant dyads, their determination to do everything possible to solve problems on their own before reaching out for help. I also find myself impatient with their difficulty with acknowledging feelings or asking for help as I know how much richer their lives could be if they were willing to be more vulnerable.

What I've Learned from Working with Ambivalent/Resistant Dyads

Working with ambivalent/resistant dyads has taught me to be more comfortable with anger and negative affect. The hyperactivation of the attachment system in these dyads is like implosion therapy for someone who leans toward dismissing—so much emotion! Coaching parents in ambivalent/resistant dyads has also helped me to understand the role of emotional outbursts in connecting. After a couple of emotion-filled coaching sessions with these dyads (typically PDI sessions), I feel connected to them in a way I don't to other families. It has given me a better understanding of how anger can be a form of connection, albeit still not my favorite way to connect.

What I've Learned from Working with Disorganized and Controlling Dyads

Visiting the unresolved attachment landscape is like visiting a war-torn country. You vacillate between sadness at what they have had to endure and awe at how they have endured it. What I've learned from working with disorganized and controlling dyads is how powerful the drive to connect is—even when connecting has led to loss or pain in the past. The power of attachment to heal and to hurt is the most important lesson I have learned from working with disorganized and controlling dyads.

Because disorganized attachment is all about anxiety and we fall into our "go to" behaviors when we're anxious, disorganized attachment has also taught me about the parts of myself I'd rather not know about—those cringeworthy moments I mentioned earlier. It has also taught me to have compassion for myself in those cringeworthy moments, in the same way I strive to have compassion for the parents and children I'm working with. There is nothing like coming face to face with the ways you act when under stress to increase your compassion for others.

Working with disorganized and controlling dyads has also taught me to be more mindful. With one particularly challenging family that had intergenerational trauma, I found myself interacting in ways that made me increasingly uncomfortable, becoming defensive, overly intellectual, and sarcastic, and trying to cover up those feelings with faux enthusiasm and positivity. I began scheduling time for yoga prior to my therapy sessions with this family. There was an immediate shift in our work together. I was able to relax in my interactions with them, stay in the moment, and attend to the moments of positive interaction and joy.

The Bottom Line

One of the most important characteristics of a therapist is the ability to stay curious and open to change. Luckily, our work with parents and young children gives us plenty of opportunities to continue to grow and change. As with parenting young children, therapeutic work with young children and their parents can be challenging—especially when we feel the need for the certitude of always knowing the right answer. But it is great work when we are willing to show up, do our best, continue to reflect, and continue to grow.

References

Bromberg, P. (1998). Speak! That I may see you: Some reflections on dissociation, reality, and psychoanalytic listening. In P. Bromberg (Ed.), *Standing in the spaces: Essays on clinical process, trauma, and dissociation*. Psychology Press.

Dozier, M., & Bernard, K. (2019). *Coaching parents of vulnerable infants: The attachment and biobehavioral catch-up approach*. The Guilford Press.

References

Dozier, M., Cue, K., & Barnett, L. (1994). Clinicians as caregivers: Role of attachment organization in treatment. *Journal of Consulting and Clinical Psychology, 62*(4), 793–800.

Miller-Bottome, M., Talia, A., Eubanks, C., Safran, J., & Muran, J. (2019). Secure in-session attachment predicts rupture resolution: Negotiating a secure base. *Psychoanalytic Psychology, 36*(2), 132–138.

Miller-Bottome, M., Talia, A., Safran, J., & Muran, J. (2017). Resolving alliance ruptures from an attachment-informed perspective. *Psychoanalytic Psychology, 35*(2), 175–183.

Talia, A., Daniel, S., Miller-Bottome, M., Brambilla, D., Miccoli, D., Safran, J., & Lingiardi, V. (2014). AAI predicts patients' in-session interpersonal behavior and discourse: A "move to the level of the relation" for attachment-informed psychotherapy research. *Attachment & Human Development, 16*(2), 192–209.

Talia, A., Miller-Bottome, M., & Daniel, S. (2015). Assessing attachment in psychotherapy: Validation study of the patient attachment coding system. *Clinical Psychology & Psychotherapy, 24*, 149–161.

Talia, A., Muzi, L., Lingiardi, V., & Taubner, S. (2020). How to be a secure base: Therapists' attachment representations and their link to attunement in psychotherapy. *Attachment & Human Development, 22*(2), 189–206.

Chapter 18
Dancing Toward Security: Adding New Steps to Your Attachment Dance

> *I don't tell my body to dance; my body tells me to dance.*
> Jasper Pelzel, age 4 (Pelzel, 2021)

I end this book with a chapter about one of my first loves, dance. This final chapter includes some thoughts on the role of movement and dance in coping with stress and healing from attachment trauma. It includes a playlist of dance songs that illustrate and summarize the core concepts of attachment-informed parent coaching.

The Power of Dance

When I think of the power of dance, I remember the session where a child "built" a piano out of blocks in front of her mother. Her mother entered the child's imaginative world and began to "play the piano" singing "do da do da do," moving her hands across the blocks while her child danced. For that moment in time, the three of us were transported—beyond the daily hassles of parenting a young child, beyond parent coaching, even beyond the ghosts in the nursery that had marred the relationship between the child and her mother. We were dancing.

Dancing has always had a special place in my heart. My first memories involve dance: the red leotard I wore to my first dance class, the "kick the ball and step on it" move I learned there, the sewing cards I did while waiting for my tap class, and the beautiful older ballerinas I watched while I waited for their class to end. My childhood dance lessons lasted for the brief period of time we lived in Derby, Kansas, when I was between the ages of four-and-a-half and five. But they left an indelible mark on my soul.

Over the past few years, I have had the opportunity to rediscover the joy I find in moving to music. At a UC Davis PCIT conference I attended, Marta Shinn led a large group of adults in *Play in Place*, part of the intervention developed by Shinn and colleagues to address childhood obesity (Shinn et al., 2017). *Play in Place* is a brief activity designed to increase physical activity in obese children by having them complete a series of basic movements to music (e.g., marching, walking, and kicking) (Taylor Lucas et al., 2015). What struck me at the conference, as I looked around the room at everyone moving with Marta Shinn to the music, was how happy everyone seemed.

This experience led me to take my first dance class in several decades. And I began incorporating dance breaks into my workshops for therapists. There was often some grumbling and self-consciousness about these dance breaks, but, just as I'd experienced when Marta Shinn got people to dance together, everyone seemed to feel happier when we danced together. The dance breaks evolved into dancing to "theme songs" for each of the different attachment strategies.

Dance as a Coping Strategy During the COVID-19 Pandemic

My response to the worldwide disorganization and trauma associated with the COVID-19 pandemic that began in 2020 was to dance more. In retrospect, I am amazed at how quickly my community of therapists and dancers came together at a time of such anxiety, trauma, and stress. It was as though we all recognized the need to harness the power of dance to cope with an experience that was literally beyond words.

Virtual Dance Parties

My friend, Tracy Vozar, put together a virtual daily dance party for parents of young children. Beginning in March 2020, every day for a half hour in the morning, parents, children, and others would log on and dance in front of their computer screens. The combination of dancing and watching young children dance calmed my nervous system in a way nothing else did during this time of relative isolation. As what we thought would be a short period of isolation extended into months, we celebrated birthdays, prom, a missed trip to Paris, and other events by dancing in front of our computer screens.

Raining Tacos by Parry Gripp (2013) became my favorite dance tune as I watched the joy of children and adults alike pretending to eat tacos falling out of the sky. It reminded me that it is a generous universe—despite the challenges being dished out to virtually everyone in the world during that period. This daily dance party continued for months until evolving into a weekly dance party for the young and the young at heart.

Sing.Play.Love.® Parties

My friends Kelly Pelzel and Anne Meeker Watson offered virtual Sing.Play.Love.® parties three times a week in April and May 2020 for the children of health-care workers at the University of Iowa Hospitals and Clinics. More information about the Sing.Play.Love.® approach and materials developed by Anne Meeker Watson is available at https://www.singplaylove.com/.

The Sing.Play.Love.® parties, scheduled in the afternoons so I didn't have to miss my morning dance parties, included reading books and sing-a-longs. The sing-a-longs incorporated activities involving both small and large motor movements. As my own travels were curtailed, I loved watching babies dancing from their mother's laps as we drove along to Woody Guthrie's *Car Song* (Guthrie, 1997). Watching parents sensitively adapt the activities for their infants was a powerful reminder of the ordinary magic of secure attachment during a time of worldwide insecurity. I experienced the power of synchronous movement as we all jumped forward together, jumped back together, and balanced on one foot—adults and children alike smiling as we sang, moved, and struggled to balance. I also experienced the power of movement and music to bring us together as we sang what I consider one of Anne Meeker Watson's greatest hits, *I Take the Music with Me* (Watson, 2019), before waving goodbye at the end of each party.

BeMoved® Dance Classes

My own contribution to connecting through dance was to offer a weekly virtual BeMoved® dance class for my aunt, Karolyn Leary, sister, Juli Troutman, and cousin, Teri McClure Elliott, beginning in March 2020. More information about the BeMoved® dance experience designed by Sherry Zunker is available at the BeMoved® website: https://bemoveddance.com/. What began as a replacement for the in-person BeMoved® dance class my aunt and I attended prior to the pandemic has become a new tradition as we continue to dance, connect, and chat once a week from different parts of the country.

I also offered virtual BeMoved® dance classes for IoWA-PCIT therapists three times a week during April and May 2020. Therapists told me they especially appreciated the stretches and shoulder rolls as we all adjusted to spending our days hunched over our computers in Zoom meetings and telehealth sessions. In addition to the joy of sharing my love of dance with others, the challenge of learning new dance steps and teaching them over Zoom provided a welcome distraction from the numerous stressors and adjustments we encountered during this period.

Born to Dance

These experiences have been so powerful that it makes me wonder what it is about dance and movement that creates such joy. Carla Mears, a student of Harry Harlow, noted that in addition to being born for relationships, we are born to move (Mears, 1978). She chose the term peragration, the motion of a body through space, to describe her observations of infant rhesus monkeys moving their bodies for no apparent reason other than the sheer joy of locomotor movement. As noted in a recent study of the peragration hypothesis, "Infant monkeys run, turn flips, and tumble with no toys, apparatus, or playmates to incite locomotion. Similarly, foals gambol, puppies chase their tails, and human infants run laps around the living room" (Hoch et al., 2019). Before we get to the results of the study, take a minute to picture baby animals moving and see if it doesn't make you smile.

Hoch et al. (2019) compared the locomotor exploration of 15-month-olds in a room filled with toys selected to encourage locomotion (e.g., a popper that pops plastic balls when rolled and a baby doll stroller) and a room with no toys. In other words, this study examined whether toddlers primarily move to get somewhere (the destination-directed hypothesis) or whether they move for the sake of movement (the peragration hypothesis). Consistent with the peragration hypothesis, the amount of locomotion did not differ between the two groups—toddlers in the room without toys covered as much ground as toddlers in the room with toys. Given room to move, young children move. They don't need any additional motivation—their body tells them to dance.

Movement and Attachment

Mary Ainsworth describes the fact that locomotion in infants coincides with the development of a strong specific attachment to caregivers as a "happy coincidence" (Ainsworth et al., 1978). She goes on to suggest that it may not be a coincidence. That is, there is an evolutionary advantage to the powerful drive to move being balanced out by an equally powerful drive to maintain proximity to parents. Once infants learn to move, movement can be used to gain and maintain proximity with their attachment figure, as well as for the sheer joy of moving. When observing mothers and infants in their homes, I was struck by how a baby who was seemingly oblivious to his mother's whereabouts as he crawled about exploring his world would immediately crawl after his mother when she left the room.

Movement in Secure Dyads

As with other aspects of how we engage in the world, how we move is impacted by our experiences in relationships. When I reflect on the movements of children in secure attachment relationships, I think about how self-assured and confident they are in their movements. I remember a 3-year-old striding confidently around the room in her cowboy boots after her mother left the room. She used all the space in the playroom—moving from one corner to the next and marching around the perimeter. Each time she got to the edge of the room, she triumphantly raised her arms to the sky before setting off again. She accompanied this confident striding with an impromptu song about her mother being gone as though she was performing in her own musical about separation.

Not every child in a secure dyad moves around the room with this type of exuberance. Others own the space in a quieter way during separations from their parents —exploring through creative play. I remember a 2-year-old using blocks to build umbrellas for the baby dolls to protect them from the rain and a 6-year-old confidently building a cityscape out of Legos. Although they explored the space in different ways, they exuded the same type of self-confidence in their motor abilities.

During the reunion with their parents, I see children in secure dyads exhibit this same confident movement whether the child has been distressed or playing contentedly during the parent's absence. The 1-year-olds frequently crawl or toddle to the door, reaching out confidently to their parent as they smile and reach for them—exhibiting the infectious joy of being able to move toward the most important person in your world.

I remember the 3-year-old who sang and danced in her own musical about separation striding confidently toward her mother when her mother returned. After greeting her mother, she skipped back to the center of the room, barely able to contain her exuberance at her mother's return and confident that her mother would follow. I remember the 2-year-old who greeted her mother from the floor, explaining to her mother how she had built umbrellas out of the blocks for the babies, and the 6-year-old who danced to the door to share her joy in the cityscape she had created during her mother's absence.

Movement in Ambivalent/Resistant Dyads

In contrast to the confident movements of children in secure dyads, I think of the hesitant, anxious movements of children in ambivalent/resistant dyads. I remember the 1-year-olds who seemed too overcome with distress during their parent's absence to use their newfound motor skills to seek their parent. I remember the 4-year-old standing in the corner during his parent's absence, rhythmically hitting the wall as he waits for his mother's return. I remember him briefly tiptoeing away from the corner—his tentative, cautious movements a stark contrast to the self-confident movements of children in secure attachment relationships.

During the reunion with the parent, I remember the difficulty in trying to make sense of the conflicted movements of children in ambivalent/resistant dyads—a painful dance in which they both seek and reject their parents. I remember the 1-year-olds who sat in the middle of the floor and cried, continuing to be upset and actively squirming when their parent picked them up when they returned. I remember the 4-year-old who tentatively took his parent's hand when she returned but seemed lost as to what to do next. I remember the 5-year-old who, after anxiously awaiting his parent's return, turned away from her when she entered the room, giving away his anxious tracking of her movements only when she briefly turned away from him and his gaze followed her.

Movement in Avoidant Dyads

When I think of movement in avoidant attachment, I remember the purposeful yet joyless movement of infants and young children in avoidant attachment relationships. I remember the 1-year-olds who move around the room examining the various toys as though they are taking inventory and who become intently interested in exploring a toy when the parent returns. I remember the 5-year-old whose movements seemed carefully choreographed to keep a certain distance from his parent during the reunion—not too close and not too far.

Movement in Disorganized Dyads

When I reflect on movement during disorganized attachment relationships, I remember the awkward movements involved in being stuck between a rock and a hard place. I remember the 1-year-old who stood crying, moved toward her parent, and then ducked under her mother's chair. I remember the 3-year-old who, after crying at the door for her mother, moved toward her, darted away, and then wandered around the room with a dazed expression. Unlike the fluid, graceful dance seen in secure attachment or the carefully choreographed dance seen in ambivalent/resistant and avoidant attachment, the dance in disorganized attachment feels unpredictable.

Movement in Controlling Dyads

When I think about movement in controlling attachment relationships, I think about how the dance is rigidly choreographed by the child. The quality of movement in controlling dyads shares the anxious quality seen in ambivalent/resistant dyads but it is anything but tentative. Children in controlling dyads lack the relaxed self-confidence seen in children in secure dyads—it is difficult for them to let their guard down and enjoy the dance. I remember the 5-year-old who immediately took charge when his parent returned, directing his parent's movements by telling her where to sit and what to do—an exacting taskmaster who seemed unable to trust his mother to make her own decisions. I also remember the 6-year-old whose dance became increasingly frenetic and lively as she attempted to cheer up her father with her dance performance. Children in controlling attachment relationships are so focused on choreographing the movement of their parent, they lack the freedom to explore their own dance.

Providing Opportunities to Dance

Luckily, everyone is born a dancer—not just those born into secure attachment relationships or with exceptional motor skills. The moments of joyful, self-confident movement that seem especially prevalent in secure dyads also occur in insecure dyads. Just as attending to the moments of secure attachment during parent coaching can remind children they are born for relationships, attending to moments of joyful movement can remind children they are born to dance.

In a study comparing the movement of preschool children in different playground environments, children engaged in more physical activity when they had open play space where they could move freely (Berg, 2015). So, make sure your playroom has plenty of room to dance and celebrate the moments where children are moving through space.

Dance Music

My friend, the brilliant music therapist Anne Meeker Watson, reminds me that part of the special healing power of dance is that it is typically accompanied by music, which has its own special magic. Since I can't literally teach you how to dance in this chapter, I will share the music of some of my favorite attachment songs. The IoWA-PCIT attachment strategies playlist in Table 18.1 lists "theme songs" for the different attachment strategies. So, take a break from reading and dance with me.

Table 18.1 IoWA-PCIT attachment strategies playlist

Secure/autonomous	*Something just like this* The Chainsmokers and Coldplay
	The age of miracles Mary Chapin Carpenter
	Think about things Daði Freyr Petursson
	Three Lily Allen
	Piece by piece Kelly Clarkson
Avoidant/dismissing	*Stronger (what doesn't kill you)* Kelly Clarkson
	I'm still standing Elton John
	People will say we're in love Oscar Hammerstein II and Richard Rodgers
Ambivalent/resistant Preoccupied	*True love* Pink, Greg Kurstin, and Lily Allen
	Hard to love Aamity Mae
Disorganized/unresolved	*Poison & wine* The Civil Wars
	Anthem Leonard Cohen
Controlling–punitive	*I hate myself for loving you* Joan Jett and Desmond Childs
Controlling–caregiving	*You are my sunshine* Jimmie Davis and Charles Mitchell

Songs for Secure Pattern of Attachment and Secure/Autonomous State of Mind

You may have noticed there are more songs for secure attachment than for any other attachment strategy. This is a reminder that most attachment relationships are secure. Or, as stated in Chap. 1, we are born for relationships.

Something Just Like This by The Chainsmokers and Coldplay illustrates the ordinariness of secure attachment (Taggart et al., 2017). I love the emphasis of the song's lyrics on not having to be a superhero in order to be a safe haven for someone. Instead, you have to be available so the other person can turn to you when they need you. When working with parents, one of our most important interventions is pointing out the "something just like this" (Taggart et al., 2017) moments they provide for their child. Sometimes when working with families, we forget that secure attachment is the norm, not the exception. Even in clinical and at-risk populations, we often encounter dyads with secure attachment relationships. And we encounter moments of security even in insecure dyads.

The Age of Miracles by Mary Chapin Carpenter illustrates the wonderful gift of having an early foundation of secure attachment (Carpenter, 2010). The first time I heard this song I was struck by the description of calamitous events and overwhelming grief. But I later heard the sense of optimism that comes from having a safe haven to return to—even if that safe haven is in memory or imagination. This song speaks to me about finding joy in the midst of sorrow and trauma and finding hope in the midst of despair. When working with young children and their parents, we can become overwhelmed with the trauma and hardships they have endured. This song reminds me to relish the courage of these families and the small miracles we are privileged to share with them.

Think About Things by Daði Freyr was written by a father about his relationship with his baby daughter (Petursson, 2020). Check out the video for killer dance moves. This song captures a new father's anxiety about his relationship with his infant daughter, his hope that he will be a safe haven for his daughter, and his fears that he won't be able to understand his daughter's cues. Thanks to Tracy Vozar for pointing me to this secure attachment song.

Three by Lily Allen (2018) is a superb example of a song that speaks for the child. Allen puts herself in her young daughter's shoes and ably describes her daughter's attachment and exploration needs. *Three* (Allen, 2018) reminds me that a parent's ability to unflinchingly recognize their child's attachment and exploration signals is a gift. This song captures both the poignant longing of young children for their parents and their ability to keep their parent in mind during separations. It also captures what children most enjoy doing with their parents—playing.

Piece by Piece by Kelly Clarkson sums up the pathway to the "earned secure" attachment state of mind for adults who had difficult relationships with parents in childhood (Clarkson, 2015). Clarkson acknowledges the pain associated with a difficult relationship with a parent and the effort to build a different type of attachment relationship. The piece missing from this song is forgiveness, which is an important part of earned security.

Songs for Avoidant Pattern of Attachment and Dismissing State of Mind

Stronger (What Doesn't Kill You) by Kelly Clarkson (2011) illustrates the avoidant strategy of relying solely on oneself to cope with distress, that is, deactivation of the attachment system. In parents with a dismissing state of mind, there is an exclusive emphasis on personal strength. Moments of vulnerability, such as when revealing situations where they were hurt or rejected by a parent, are immediately followed by a positive wrap-up about how this resulted in them being tougher.

Stronger (What Doesn't Kill You) (Clarkson, 2011) illustrates why parents with a dismissing state of mind may be experienced by therapists as resistant and combative. The song points out the strategy of becoming a fighter in response to hardship.

So, when you're dancing to Kelly Clarkson's *Stronger* video, remember how great it feels to be confident and powerful (the choreography helps with this feeling). Remember that feeling when you are working with parents who are resistant and combative. And also remember that this strategy of response to authority figures likely developed out of the parent's experience of their own parents as rejecting, neglectful, and/or unresponsive to distress, which is how they are likely to experience you and others.

I'm Still Standing by Elton John and Bernie Taupin illustrates how deactivation of the attachment system is a strategy that works when parents are limited in their ability to meet the child's attachment needs (John & Taupin, 1983). The brilliance of this song is that it also gives us a glimpse into the vulnerability behind this attachment strategy. My favorite music video for *I'm Still Standing* is from the movie *Sing*. This music video illustrates the deep love of Johnny's father for his son, despite the father's failure to recognize and meet his son's needs for acknowledgment. When working with parents with a more dismissing attachment state of mind who want to "toughen up" their children so they can cope with a harsh world, it can be difficult to recognize this as love. Like other parents with dismissing attachment, Johnny's father clearly loves his son. This song reminds us of the importance of helping dismissing parents find a better way of expressing this love. Thanks to Sarah Taber-Thomas for pointing me to this song and music video as an example of avoidant and dismissing attachment.

People Will Say We're in Love from the musical *Oklahoma!* (Hammerstein II & Rodgers, 1943) is an example of avoidant attachment moving toward security. This is best illustrated in the version performed by Damon Daunno and Rebecca Naomi Jones in the 2019 revival of *Oklahoma!* where Daunno and Jones literally move toward each other during the song (https://www.broadwayworld.com/videoplay/VIDEO-Damon-Daunno-and-Rebecca-Naomi-Jones-Perform-from-OKLAHOMA-20190531). As with many dyads we see with avoidant attachment, at the beginning of the song in the musical, the characters primarily express their attachment needs through a series of prohibitions—telling each other all the things they need to avoid doing in order to keep others from noticing their feelings for each other. By the end of the song, they have become secure enough in their attachment to want to share their feelings with the world—even praising each other by the end of the song.

Songs for Ambivalent/Resistant Pattern of Attachment and Preoccupied State of Mind

True Love by Alecia Moore (Pink), Greg Kurstin, and Lily Allen (2013) illustrates the attachment strategy for individuals in ambivalent/resistant attachment relationships. This strategy for being in relationships is at the other end of the spectrum from avoidant. The ambivalent/resistant attachment strategy is characterized by an intense focus on attachment relationships accompanied by intense anger and ambivalence about these relationships. This is referred to as hyperactivation of the attachment system. When working with such parent–child dyads, therapists may be baffled by the combination of the child's intense distress at separation and anger and aggression toward the parent at the reunion. *True Love* (Moore et al., 2013) describes the intense need for physical closeness and attachment mixed with feelings of wanting to hurt the attachment figure. This song captures the child's experience of being in an ambivalent/resistant dyad; being angry at the parent but having no other option for getting their attachment needs met.

True Love (Moore et al., 2013) also captures the way individuals with a preoccupied working model of attachment focus on the ways they have been wronged in attachment relationships, even as they remain enmeshed in those relationships. Parents with a preoccupied working model of attachment may be experienced by therapists as needy and dramatic. It helps to remember that this strategy developed out of the parent's experience of their own parents being inconsistent, which is how they are likely to experience therapists.

Hard to Love by Aamity Mae (2016) describes the excitement of being in the type of intense relationship characterized by hyperactivation of the attachment system. *Hard to Love* (Mae, 2016) captures the drama of being in a demanding relationship—and the ambivalence about being in a relationship that was less fraught. *Hard to Love* (Mae, 2016) also describes the downside of ambivalent/resistant attachment relationships—the difficulty of interpreting the mixed signals of individuals in these dyads. This song also captures the countertransference experience of therapists working with ambivalent/resistant dyads, that is, the therapist's painful realization that it could be difficult to love either the child or the parent in the dyad.

Songs for Disorganized Pattern of Attachment and Unresolved State of Mind

Poison & Wine by The Civil Wars (Williams & White, 2009) captures how painful it is to be in a disorganized attachment relationship. For children who lack an organized attachment strategy with their parent, the parent is both the safe haven and the source of anxiety. This leaves the child in a disorganized attachment relationship stuck between a rock and a hard place. This song speaks to how much the child in a disorganized attachment relationship loves their parent—even as the child attempts to resolve their dilemma by not loving the parent. The child's experience of not being seen or understood by their attachment figure—the failure that is ultimately at the root of disorganized attachment—is captured by this song. Whether because of the parent's own unresolved loss or attachment trauma, the parent is unable to put themselves in the child's shoes—which may ultimately be the most damaging aspect of disorganized attachment. As therapists, our goal is to help parents in disorganized attachment relationships see their child and be able to understand their child's perspective. By helping the parent understand the impact of their behavior on their child, we decrease the toxic interactions that keep the child from reliably using their parent as a secure base and safe haven.

As *Anthem* by Leonard Cohen (1992) evokes, healing from disorganized attachment and unresolved traumatic attachment experiences involves learning to live in the moment. *Anthem* (Cohen, 1992) reminds me that showing up and witnessing is an important part of what I do in working with disorganized and unresolved attachment—perhaps the most important part. It also reminds me to embrace the messy imperfection in being human.

Song for Controlling–Punitive Attachment

I Hate Myself for Loving You by Joan Jett and Desmond Child (1988) captures the anger of being in an attachment relationship where you are trying to rely on someone who is unreliable. It speaks to the anxiety underlying the anger we see in controlling–punitive attachment relationships. It is often difficult to be empathetic with children in a controlling–punitive attachment relationship—it is tough to like someone who is just so mean to their parent. *I Hate Myself for Loving You* (Jett & Child, 1988) helps us understand the core of the child's anger—the child is angry at themselves and their own attachment needs. The spiteful way the child is controlling their parent is an indication of how much the child desperately needs their parent's love. It is this very desperation that leads them to try to control interactions with their parent. So, next time you're frustrated with coaching a controlling–punitive dyad, dance to some Joan Jett before the session. I know you can't stay angry at Joan. Let her lyrics remind you of how hard it is for the child to have to be in control to get their attachment needs met. And remember how lucky the child is to have you and Joan on their side.

Song for Controlling–Caregiving Attachment

You Are My Sunshine by Jimmie Davis and Charles Mitchell (1940) captures the controlling–caregiving strategy for maintaining a relationship with an unreliable caregiver. For me, *You Are My Sunshine* (Davis & Mitchell, 1940) captures the complicated combination of feelings in controlling–caregiving dyads: the heady feeling of being so important to someone else that their life depends on it *and* the feelings of sadness and anxiety that accompany that role. One of the characteristics of children in a controlling–caregiving dyad is their overbright smile, an indication of how hard they are trying to cheer up and take care of their parent. As with other disorganized dyads, at the heart of this dyad is a parent so overwhelmed by their own grief or attachment trauma they are unable to recognize their child's needs.

The Bottom Line

Throughout this book, I have talked about the special dance we are involved in when doing parent coaching—following the steps of the parent and child until we understand their dance well enough to teach them a few new steps. I leave you with a song that illustrates our most important contribution as attachment-informed therapists, *The Nearness of You* by Hoagy Carmichael and Ned Washington (1940). There are so many beautiful covers of this song it is difficult to choose a favorite. I suggest picking a cover by Norah Jones, Nicole Henry, or James Taylor.

The lyrics of this song remind us that our healing relationship with parents and children—witnessing and providing a holding environment for them as they struggle and grow—is a critical piece of our work with families. After dancing my way through attachment workshops by using songs to illustrate attachment strategies, I felt I had discovered a kindred spirit when Philip Bromberg (2011) quoted *The Nearness of You* (Carmichael & Washington, 1940) in *The Shadow of the Tsunami and the Growth of the Relational Mind*, to illustrate what it is like to be in the presence of someone who gets you in a deep way. Being seen and understood deeply is the core aspect of our most important and healing relationships (Bromberg, 2011).

As a therapist, the most important gift you can give the parents you're coaching is your nearness—not what you say, not what you do, just being near them as they find new ways to connect with their child. Your nearness helps parents recognize an important truth—their presence is the most important thing in the world to their child.

References

Ainsworth, M., Blehar, M., Waters, E., & Wall, S. (1978). *Patterns of attachment: A psychological study of the strange situation*. Erlbaum.
Allen, L. (2018). Three. On *No shame*.
Berg, S. (2015). Children's activity levels in different playground environments: An observational study in four Canadian preschools. *Early Childhood Education Journal, 43*, 281–287.
Bromberg, P. (2011). *The shadow of the tsunami and the growth of the relational mind*. Taylor & Francis Group, LLC.
Carmichael, H., & Washington, N. (1940). Famous music.
Carpenter, M. C. (2010). The age of miracles. On *The age of miracles*. Zoe Records.
Clarkson, K. (2011). Stronger (what doesn't kill you). On *Stronger*. RCA Records.
Clarkson, K. (2015). Piece by piece. On *Piece by piece*. RCA Records.
Cohen, L. (1992). *Anthem*. Sony.
Davis, J., & Mitchell, C. (1940). *You are my sunshine*. Southern Music Publishing Co..
Gripp, P. (2013). Raining tacos. On *Mega-party*. Parry Gripp Records.
Guthrie, W. (1997). Car song. On *This land is your land: The Asch recordings, Volume 1*.
Hammerstein II, O., & Rodgers, R. (1943). On *Oklahoma!* People Will Say We're in Love, Decca Records, Kensington, London, United Kingdom.
Hoch, J., O'Grady, S., & Adolph, K. (2019). It's the journey, not the destination: Locomotor exploration in infants. *Developmental Science, 22*(2), e12740.
Jett, J., & Child, D. (1988). I hate myself for loving you. On *Up your alley*. Blackheart.
John, E., & Taupin, B. (1983). I'm still standing. *Too low for zero*. Geffen.

Mae, A. (2016). Hard to love. On *AamityMae*.
Mears, C. (1978). Play and development of cosmic confidence. *Developmental Psychology, 14*(4), 371–378.
Moore, A., Kurstin, G., & Allen, L. (2013). True love. On *The truth about love*. RCA Records.
Petursson, D. F. (2020). *Think about things*. AWAL.
Shinn, M., Timmer, S., & Sandoz, T. (2017). Coaching to improve mealtime parenting in treating pediatric obesity. *Clinical Practice in Pediatric Psychology, 5*(3), 232–247.
Taggart, A., Martin, C., Berryman, G., Buckland, J., & Champion, W. (2017). Something just like this. On *Memories ... do not open*. Columbia.
Taylor Lucas, C. E., Shinn, M., & Turner, A. (2015). *Play in place*. Mike Irwin Studios.
Watson, A. M. (2019). I take the music with me.
Williams, J., & White, J. (2009). Poison & wine. On *Live at Eddie's Attic: The civil wars*. Decatur, Georgia.

Index

A
Adoptive families, 158
Adult Attachment Interview (AAI), 22, 26, 27, 49, 85, 88, 99, 135, 138, 162, 163, 165
Adult-size chair, 55
Ainsworth, M., 3, 7, 20, 25, 48, 49, 55, 73, 74, 77, 91, 92, 97, 155
Altruism, 4, 5, 36
Ambivalent/resistant attachment, 7
    adaptive for the child, 94
    course of IoWA-PCIT, 96
    development of attachment pattern, 92–94
    prevalence, 94
    recognition, 91–92
    resistance, 92
    secure attachment, 94–96
    types, 92
Ambivalent/resistant dyads, 167, 175, 176
Ambivalent/resistant parent–child attachment relationship, 69
Ambivalent/resistant pattern songs
    Hard to Love, 181
    True Love, 180, 181
Anxiety, 47, 68–71, 131, 132
Anxiety-provoking, 93
Attachment
    avoidant/dismissing working model, 68
    IoWA-PCIT, 64–71
    parent's working model, 71
Attachment and adoption relationship
    adopted and biological children, 156
    adoptive parents, 157
    assessment, 156
    CDI coaching, 157
    child's behavioral/emotional problems, 156
    circumstances associated, 156
    discrepancy, 156
    loss/trauma, 157
    maltreatment, 157
    nonadopted children, 156
    parents, adopted children, 156
    PDI, 158
    psychoeducation, 156
    seasonal changes indicators, 157
    secure working model, 157
Attachment and biobehavioral catch-up (ABC), 32
Attachment anxiety, 140
Attachment assessment, 19, 25
Attachment-based home-visiting intervention, 86, 88
Attachment cues, 10–13, 79
Attachment–exploration balance, 91, 109
Attachment-informed approach, 161
Attachment-informed assessment, 20
Attachment-informed parent coaching, 65, 143, 158, 164
    approach, 10, 11, 15, 16
    biological parents, 151, 152
    child gradual exposure, 152
    child–parent relationship, 151
    physical abuse/neglect, 152
    PRIDE skills, 152
    TF-CBT, 152
Attachment-informed therapists, 183
Attachment patterns, 124
Attachment person, 10
Attachment priming, 5–6, 119
Attachment relationship disorganization, 125

Attachment security priming, 5
Attachment signals, 76–80
Attachment strategy, 128
Attachment system, deactivation, 109, 111
Attachment theory, 10, 12, 13, 16, 26, 33, 123
    Ainsworth, Mary, 3
    Bowlby, John, 2
    development, 3
    insecure attachment, 6
    parent–child relationships, 6
    principles, 1
    research, 2
Attachment trauma
    multiple layers, 143
    psychoanalytic patients, 145
    relationship, 145
    young children, 145
    young children in foster care, 143
Autonomous-secure AAIs, 49
Avoidant attachment, 6, 68, 110, 176, 180
    adaptive for the child, 111
    attachment–exploration balance, 109
    course of IoWA-PCIT with avoidant dyads, 112–113
    development, 110
    dyads, 109, 110
    parents of children, 110
    pattern, 109
    prevalence, 110
    secure attachment in avoidant dyads, 111–112
Avoidant dyads, 109, 167
Avoidant pattern songs
    I'm Still Standing, 180
    People Will Say We're in Love, 180
    Stronger (What Doesn't Kill You), 179, 180

B
Backup consequence, 57
Beebe, B., 91, 93, 135, 138
Behavioral assessment, 19, 25, 26
Behavioral parent coaching model, 9, 11
Behavior description, 34, 35, 39, 44, 45
BeMoved® dance classes, 173
Biological parents, 155
Born to play, 31, 32
Bowlby, J., 2–4
Bowlby's trilogy, 123
Bromberg, P., 21, 28
Bucharest Early Intervention Project, 143

C
Careful assessment, 20
CDI coaching, 67–69, 94, 95, 97
    in family's home, 44–45
    goal and attending, 42
    observations, 42
    psychoanalytic play therapy, 42
    sessions, 34
    statements, 42
    tracking progress, 42–44
CDI engage and teach session, 33, 34
CDI homework, 40, 41
CDI phase, 45
CDI with foster parents
    children embarrassment, 148
    child's experience, 149
    child's traumatic play, 148
    experiences, 148
    experiential reminder, 149
    feelings of distress, 148
    opportunity, 148
    real-life dangerous/destructive behavior, 149
Chase and dodge dynamic, 93
Child and Adolescent Psychiatry division, 15
Child-Directed Interaction (CDI), 13, 49, 81, 112, 113, 118, 120, 121, 130, 133, 139, 157, 164
Child-Directed Interaction (CDI) skills, 65, 67
    coaching (*see* CDI coaching)
    engage and teach session, 33, 34
    homework, 40, 41
    IoWA-PCIT, 32
    managing behavior problems, 39–40
    managing child's behavior outside, 41, 42
    parent nonverbal behaviors, 37, 38
    parent verbalizations, 34–37
    parent verbalizations avoided, 38–39
    rules and structure, 32, 33
Childhood traumatic experiences, 145
Child-led play
    benefits, 32
    born to play, 31, 32
    CDI (*see* Child-Directed Interaction (CDI) skills)
    type, 39
Child–parent interactions, 133
Child–Parent Psychotherapy (CPP), 32, 111
Child–parent relationship, 16, 156
Children in securely attached dyads, 78
Child's attachment cues, 79, 80, 82

Index 187

Child's attachment signals, 32
Child's behavior, 27, 39, 48
Child's disruptive behavior, 164
Child's intrinsic motivation, 37
Child's lead, 60
Child's pattern of attachment, 23
Child's social-emotional functioning, 36
Child's strategy, 25
Child's working model, 27
Circle of Security, 137
Coaching parents, 64, 99, 100, 102
Coaching PDI, 55
Commands, 38
Committed compliance, 52
Compliance
   committed, 52
   and noncompliance (*see* Noncompliance)
   PDI (*see* Parent-Directed
      Interaction (PDI))
   reason before command and/or after
      compliance, 51
   response to, 54
   and set limits, 47
Controlled exposure, 137
Controlling attachment
   adaptive, 129
   attachment relationship, 126, 127
   controlling behavior, 126
   controlling–caregiving, 127
   controlling–punitive relationship, 127
   development, 127, 128
   prevalence, 129
   recognize, 126
Controlling behavior, 126
Controlling–caregiving attachment, 127–129
Controlling–caregiving attachment song, 182
Controlling–caregiving behaviors, 128
Controlling–caregiving strategy, 131, 182
Controlling child–parent dyads, 123
Controlling dyads, 168, 176, 177
Controlling–punitive, 127
Controlling–punitive attachment, 127
Controlling–punitive attachment songs, 182
Controlling–punitive strategy, 131
Controlling strategy, 131
Course of IoWA-PCIT
   with earned secure parents, 88–89
   with secure/autonomous parents, 88
COVID-19 pandemic, 44, 45
Criticism, 38

D
Dance
   movements, 171
   music, 177
   opportunities, 177
   theme songs, 172
Dance as coping strategy, COVID-19
      pandemic
   BeMoved® dance class, 173
   response, 172
   Sing.Play.Love.® parties, 173
   virtual dance parties, 172
Dancing, 171
Deactivation of the attachment system, 109,
      111, 116, 121
Delight, 37
Destination-directed hypothesis, 174
Differential attention, 40
Differential reinforcement of other behavior
      (DRO), 14
Discipline, 47, 49, 57
Discrepancies, 27, 28
Dismissing attachment, 68, 71, 180
   adaptive strategy, 116–117
   in ambivalent/resistant relationship with
      their child, 120–121
   course of IoWA-PCIT with dismissing
      parents, 117–120
   description, 115
   group of individuals, 116
   prevalence, 117
   in secure relationship with their child, 120
Dismissing therapists, 164, 165
Disorganized and controlling dyads, 131, 132
Disorganized attachment, 176, 181
   adaptive, 128
   anxiety, 168
   cumulative stress, 125
   loss, 123–125
   parents' frightened behavior, 125, 126
   parents' frightening behavior, 125
   prevalence, 129
   recognize, 126
   relationships, 133
Disorganized/controlling child–parent
      attachment relationship, 71
Disorganized/disoriented attachment, 7
Disorganized pattern songs
   Anthem, 182
   Poison & Wine, 181

Disorganized spiral, 131
Disorganizing loss and trauma, 123
Disruptive behavior, 20, 23
   and aggression, 10
   children, 10
   evidence-based approaches, 9
   improvements, 15
   operant conditioning principles, 9
   parent ratings, 14, 43
   parenting factors, 14
   residential setting, 10
Drawing, 36
Dyadic Parent–Child Interaction Coding System (DPICS), 14, 19, 25, 26, 43, 125
Dymphna van den Boom research, 10

E
Early-childhood experiences, 166
Early-childhood interventionists, 21
Early-childhood mental health, 19, 20, 29
Earned secure attachment, 85, 86, 88
Earned secure working model of attachment, 86
Earned security, 179
Emotion-filled coaching sessions, 167
Empathy, 21
Enjoy, 37, 38
Enjoyment, 37
Evidence-based approaches, 9
Evidence-based interventions, 11
Exposure therapy, 137
Eyberg Child Behavior Inventory (ECBI), 14, 23, 43, 61

F
Face-to-face interactions, 93
Faux enthusiasm, 168
Filial Play Therapy, 32
Foster care, 10, 11, 146
Foster parents challenges, 146–148
"Forever home", 158

G
Gray, P., 31, 32

H
Handrails, 55
Hanf's parent coaching model, 9

Happy coincidence, 174
Harlow, H., 3
Healthy attachment, limit-setting, 48, 49
Here-and-now' skills, 86
Hyperactivation, 91, 100, 101, 104, 167

I
Imitation, 37
Individual psychotherapy, 136
Individuals with dismissing attachment, 115, 116
Infancy in Uganda (book), 155
Infant and early-childhood mental health assessment, 19
Infants, 1, 22
   in ambivalent/resistant attachment relationships, 7
   attachment relationship, 6
   attachment theory, 3
   misdirected movements, 7
   patterns of attachment, 6
   and young children, 22
Initial in-session PDI commands, 59
Initial intake, IoWA-PCIT, 23, 24
Initial PDI session, 57
Insecure attachment, 6, 7, 156
Insecure working models, 162
In-session balance between PDI and CDI, 60
Integration of Working Model of Attachment into Parent–Child Interaction Therapy (IoWA-PCIT), 9, 49, 50, 55, 64–66, 69–71, 73, 79, 81, 82
   attachment assessment, 25
   behavioral assessment, 25, 26
   CDI, 32, 130
   child–parent relationship, 130
   child's experience, 131
   clues, 26–28
   disorganized and controlling dyads, 130
   disorganized attachment, 131
   goals of attachment-informed assessment, 20
   initial assessment, 19
   initial intake, 23, 24
   loss/trauma, 130
   parent's internal working models of attachment, 21–23
   PDI, 47
   phases of, 49
   Preschool Strange Situation Procedure, 19
   pretreatment assessment, 24
   pretreatment mental health assessment, 19

reducing disruptive behavior, 132
in relationship context, 19, 20
sessions, 132
trauma-informed intervention, 130
therapeutic alliance, 20, 21
Interventions associated with resolution, unresolved attachment
    Circle of Security, 137
    exposure therapy, 137
    individual psychotherapy, 136
    mentalization-based therapy, 137
    parent coaching, 137
Inventive strategy, 56
IoWA-PCIT attachment strategies, 177, 178
IoWA-PCIT coaching, 13, 140, 163
IoWA-PCIT model, 166
    ambivalent/resistant pattern, 12
    attachment theory, 12
    avoidant pattern of attachment, 12
    behaviorism, 12
    development, 10–12
    emotional regulation, 13
    insecure attachment, 13
    parent–child dyads, 12
    parent–child interactions, 12
    protocol, 13
    traditional PCIT adaptation, 13
IoWA-PCIT research
    attachment and behavioral assessments association, 14
    children with attachment challenges, 15
    clinical experience, 15, 16
    disruptive behavior changes, 15
    disruptive behavior improvements, 15
    DPICS, 14
    ECBI, 14
    PACS and PARS, 14
    parenting factors, 14
    security of attachment, 15
IoWA-PCIT therapists, 163
IoWA-PCIT training, 16

J
Jingle machine, 36

L
Labeled praise, 34–37, 44, 45
Language, 1, 3
Legal decisions, 158
Limit-setting

in healthy attachment, 48, 49
and secure attachment, 49, 50
Locomotor exploration, 174
Longitudinal study, 49
Low-stress situation, 37

M
Main, M., 85, 86, 91, 92, 115, 116
Managing behavior problems, CDI
    child's behavior, 39
    differential attention, 40
    stopping, 40
Managing child's behavior outside of CDI, 41, 42
Marino, G., 135, 138
Masten, A., 78
Mental health problems, 19
Mental health professionals, 138
Mentalization, 137
Mentalization-based therapy, 137
Miller-Bottome, M., 86, 87, 99, 118, 162
Mother–infant interaction study, 123
Movement and attachment
    ambivalent/resistant dyads, 175, 176
    avoidant dyads, 176
    caregivers, 174
    controlling dyads, 176, 177
    disorganized dyads, 176
    secure dyads, 175
Musical *Oklahoma!*, 180
Music therapist, 177

N
The Nearness of You (song), 183
Negative attention-seeking behavior, 11, 13, 33
Neglect, 145–147, 152
Noncompliance, 55
    response to, 54–56
Nondirective and psychoanalytic play therapy, 36

O
Observation strategy, 25
Older children and adolescents in foster care system, 152, 153
Out of the Toolbox: Toddlers Differentiate Wobbly and Wooden Handrails, 55
"Overbright" smile, 127

P

Parent–child dyad, 10
Parent–child interactions, 6, 7, 20, 29, 43, 44, 61, 75, 102
Parent–Child Interaction Therapy (PCIT), 9, 12, 33, 63, 64
Parent–child play, 35
Parent coaching, 23, 64, 65, 73, 79–80, 86, 95, 112, 115, 119, 137, 153
   attachment-informed approach, 161
   disorganizing moments, 166
   intervention for irritable infants, 111
   stressful moments, 164
Parent–Directed Interaction (PDI), 14, 65, 67, 70, 71, 88, 89, 95, 97, 113, 120, 139, 158, 164
   age-appropriate command, 51
   calm and courteous command, 52
   to child
      coaching parent through explanation, 57–59
      therapist explanation, 59
   clear command, 53
   compliance (*see* Compliance)
   development, 48
   enough commands, 53, 54
   individual command, 53
   initial in-session PDI commands, 59
   in-session balance between PDI and CDI, 60
   IoWA-PCIT, 47, 50
   limit-setting
      in healthy attachment, 48, 49
      and secure attachment, 49, 50
   play commands, 59, 60
   positively state the command, 50
   protocol and coaching, 47
   real commands, 60
   reason before command/after compliance, 51
   response to compliance, 54
   response to noncompliance, 54–56
   rolled out, 61
   specific skills, 47
   tell, don't ask, 52
   time-out chair, 56–57
   tracking progress, 61
   VIPP-SD, 48
Parenting strategies, 22
Parent nonverbal behaviors, CDI
   enjoy, 37, 38
   imitation, 37
Parent-only sessions, 140

Parent ratings of disruptive behavior, 43
Parents' attachment system, 137
Parents' caregiver, 128
Parents' internal working models of attachment, 21–23
Parents' investment, 22
Parents' reflective functioning, 28
Parents' sensitive responsiveness, 147
Parent—structuring, 128
Parents' verbalizations, 11
Parents' with secure/autonomous attachment, 86
Parents' with secure/autonomous state of mind, 86, 88
Parents' working model, 163
Parent verbalizations avoided during CDI
   commands, 38
   criticism, 38
   questions, 39
Parent verbalizations, CDI
   behavior description, 35
   child's behavior, 34
   labeled praise, 35–37
   reflection, 35
Passive-aggressive personality, 97
Passivity, 97
Patient's working model of attachment, 162
Pattern of attachment, 73, 78, 79
PCIT for Traumatized Children protocol (PCIT-TC), 11, 57
PCIT protocols, 11, 57
PCIT training and research program, 11
PDI protocols, 57
PDI rolled out, 61
PDI script, 56
PDI with foster parents
   disruptive behavior and aggression, 150
   maltreated and experienced attachment disruptions, 149
   maltreatment history, 150
   opportunity, 150
   predictability, 150
   standard procedure and modifications, 150
   standard protocol, 150
   subsequent sessions, 150
   traumatic memories, 149
Peragration hypothesis, 174
Plastic infant seat, 80
Platinum rule, 22
Play
   born to, 31
   characteristics, 31
   child-led play (*see* Child-led play)

commands in PCIT, 59, 60
  feature of, 32
Play in Place, 171
Playroom, 36
Play therapy, 32, 36, 41
"Play with your child", 33
Please get off the chair, 60
Please sit in the chair, 60
Pop quiz question, 39
Positive attention, 27
Positive opposites, 35
Positive physical touch, 95, 96
Positive reinforcement, 131
Post-traumatic stress disorder (PTSD), 69
Power of dance, 171, 172
Praise, 34–37, 112
Praise, Reflect, Imitate, Describe, and Enjoy (PRIDE) skills, 33, 43, 44, 152
Preoccupied attachment, 69, 181
  AAI, 99
  course of IoWA-PCIT with preoccupied parents, 100–103
  labeled preoccupied, 99
  prevalence, 100
  subtypes, 99
Preoccupied parent
  in avoidant relationship with their child, 107
  in secure relationship with their child, 107
Preoccupied patients, 99, 100
Preoccupied therapists, 165
Preoccupied working model of attachment
  adaptive, 100
  recognition, 99–100
Preschool-aged children, 1
Preschool Attachment Classification System (PACS), 14
Preschool Attachment Rating Scales (PARS), 14
Preschool Strange Situation Procedure, 19, 25
Pretreatment assessment, 20, 24, 34
Prosocial behavior, 36
Psychoanalytic play therapy, 36, 42
Psychoeducation, 155
Psychological parent, 1
Punitive and coercive techniques, 49

R
Raining Tacos by Parry, 172
Reactive attachment disorder, 15, 156
Real commands, 60
Reflection, 34, 35, 39, 44, 45

Reflective functioning, 28
Reflective supervision, 166
Regular CDI, 149
Rewards, 36
Robertson, James, 124
Robertson, Joyce, 124
Robertsons' observations, 124
Ruptures in relationships, 86, 87

S
Safe and effective consequence, 56
Secure attachment, 6, 7, 66, 76, 155–158, 163, 178
  in CDI, 95
  clear communication of attachment needs, 74
  general characteristics, 73
  haven of safety, 73
  in infants, 80–81
  in infant strange situation procedure, 74–75
  and limit-setting, 49, 50
  preschool-aged children, 74
  in preschool strange situation procedure, 76
  secure base, 74
  in toddlers and preschool-aged children, 81
Secure/autonomous attachment
  adaptive, 86–87
  prevalence, 88
  working model, 85–86
Secure child–parent attachment
  relationships, 73, 77
  signals, 76–77
Secure dyads, 167
Securely attached individuals, 87
Secure pattern songs
  Piece by Piece, 179
  Something Just Like This, 178
  The Age of Miracles, 179
  Think About Things, 179
  Three, 179
Secure therapists, 163
Self-consciousness, 172
Sensitive discipline, 48
Sensitive responsiveness, 49
  to attachment signals, 79–80
  definition, 77
Sensitive therapists, 21
Separation impacts, 124
Separation–reunion procedure, 25
Sheila Eyberg, 32, 43
Sing.Play.Love.® parties, 173

Social-emotional development, 2–3, 7
Social reinforcers, 37
Stopping CDI, 40
Strange Situation Procedure, 25, 74–76, 123, 126, 156, 157
Stress, 47

T
Talia, A., 86, 87, 99, 100, 116–119, 162–165
Teachable moments, 49
Therapeutic alliance, 19–21, 24, 87, 163
Therapeutic relationship, 161
Therapist Attunement Scales (TASc), 162
Therapist explanation, 59
Therapists
　authority, 56
　CDI engage and teach session, 34
　self-disclosure, 161
Therapist's working model of attachment
　AAI, 162, 164
　communication, 162, 163, 165
　patient's feelings, 164
　secure, 163
Time-out chair, 48, 54–59
Toddlers, 1, 5
Tracking progress
　in CDI
　　assessments and observations, 42
　　observations of parent–child interactions, 43, 44
　　parent ratings of disruptive behavior, 43
　in PDI, 61
Traditional PCIT, 11, 12, 63
Trauma-Focused Cognitive Behavioral Therapy (TF-CBT), 152
Traumatic attachment experiences, 157
Treatment approaches, 131
Treatment with parents, unresolved attachment
　behind-the-mirror coaching, 139
　CDI, 139
　IoWA-PCIT response, 138
　parent-only sessions, 140
　PDI, 139
　therapeutic relationship, 138
　time-out procedure, 139

U
Unresolved attachment, 71
　adaptive, 136
　development, 136
　interventions associated with resolution, 136–138
　landscape, 168
　loss/trauma
　　parent coaching adaptation, 135
　　recognition, 135
　prevalence, 138
　treatment with parents (*see* Treatment with parents, unresolved attachment)
Unresolved attachment trauma, 137, 138, 140
Unresolved state of mind, 71

V
Video-feedback Intervention to promote Positive Parenting and Sensitive Discipline (VIPP-SD), 48
Virginia Axline's classic text, 36
Virtual daily dance parties, 172

W
WACB-N, 61
Watch, Wait and Wonder (WWW), 32
Weekly Assessment of Child Behavior–Positive (WACB-P), 43
Winnicott, D.W., 124, 127
Working model of attachment, 161, 162

Y
Young children in foster care
　attachment myth, 144, 145
　biological parents, 151
　challenges, 143, 144
　healing, 146
　sensitively responsive parents, 153

The manufacturer's authorised representative in the EU is Springer Nature Customer Service Centre GmbH, Europaplatz 3, 69115 Heidelberg, Germany. If you have any concerns regarding our products, please contact ProductSafety@springernature.com

Printed and bound by CPI Group (UK) Ltd, Croydon, CR0 4YY

25/03/2026

02078174-0005